Jewish and Catholic Bioethics:

An Ecumenical Dialogue

MORAL TRADITIONS & MORAL ARGUMENTS
A SERIES EDITED BY JAMES F. KEENAN, S.J.

The Evolution of Altruism and the Ordering of Love
STEPHEN J. POPE

Love, Human and Divine: The Heart of Christian Ethics
EDWARD COLLINS VACEK, S.J.

Bridging the Sacred and the Secular:
Selected Writings of John Courtney Murray, S.J.
J. LEON HOOPER, S.J., editor

The Context of Casuistry
JAMES F. KEENAN, S.J. and THOMAS A. SHANNON, editors

Aquinas and Empowerment: Classical Ethics for Ordinary Lives
G. SIMON HARAK, S.J., editor

The Christian Case for Virtue Ethics
JOSEPH J. KOTVA, JR.

Feminist Ethics and Natural Law: The End of Anathemas
CRISTINA L. H. TRAINA

The Origins of Moral Theology in the United States
CHARLES E. CURRAN

The Catholic Moral Tradition Today: A Synthesis
CHARLES E. CURRAN

The Banality of Good and Evil:
Moral Lessons from the Shoah and Jewish Tradition
DAVID R. BLUMENTHAL

Jewish and Catholic Bioethics:
An Ecumenical Dialogue

EDITED BY

EDMUND D. PELLEGRINO *and* ALAN I. FADEN

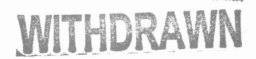

GEORGETOWN UNIVERSITY PRESS / WASHINGTON, D.C.

Georgetown University Press, Washington, D.C.
© 1999 by Georgetown University Press. All rights reserved.
Printed in the United States of America

10   9   8   7   6   5   4   3   2   1   1999

THIS VOLUME IS PRINTED ON ACID-FREE OFFSET BOOK PAPER

Library of Congress Cataloging-in-Publication Data

Jewish and Catholic bioethics : an ecumenical dialogue / edited by
    Edmund D. Pellegrino and Alan I. Faden.
        p.   cm.—(Moral traditions & moral arguments series)
    Includes index.
    ISBN 0-87840-745-6 (cloth). — ISBN 0-87840-746-4 (paper)
    1. Bioethics—Religious aspects—Judaism. 2. Medicine—Religious
aspects—Judaism. 3. Suffering—Religious aspects—Judaism.
4. Ethics, Jewish. I. Pellegrino, Edmund D., 1920–   . II. Faden,
Alan I.
R725.57.J45   1999
296.3′642—DC21
                                                    99-12407
                                                    CIP

Contents

Acknowledgment

The authors gratefully acknowledge the invaluable assistance of Clementine C. Pellegrino, M.S.L.S., and David G. Miller, M.A., for their editing, checking bibliographic references, and reconciling texts. Without their help, the usual complexities of a multi-authored work would have been much more difficult to negotiate.

Contributors

TOM L. BEAUCHAMP, PH.D.   Professor of Philosophy, Senior Research Scholar, Kennedy Institute of Ethics, Georgetown University, Washington, D.C.

BARUCH A. BRODY, PH.D.   Leon Jaworski Professor of Biomedical Ethics; Director, Center for Medical Ethics and Health Policy, Baylor College of Medicine; Professor of Medicine, Rice University, Houston, Texas

REV. JOSEPH DANIEL CASSIDY, O.P., PH.D.   Special Lecturer in Philosophy, Providence College, Providence, Rhode Island

ALAN I. FADEN, M.D.   Professor, Georgetown Institute for Cognitive and Computational Sciences, Georgetown University Medical Center, Washington, D.C.

SHIMON GLICK, M.D.   The Gussie Krupp Professor of Internal Medicine, Ben Gurion University of the Negev, Be'ér Shéva', Israel

RONALD M. GREEN, PH.D.   Director, Institute for the Study of Applied and Professional Ethics, Dartmouth College, Hanover, New Hampshire

REV. JAMES KEENAN, S.J.   Professor, Weston Jesuit College of Theology, Cambridge, Massachusetts

EDMUND D. PELLEGRINO, M.D., M.A.C.P.   The John Carroll Professor of Medicine and Medical Ethics; Director, Center for Clinical Bioethics, Georgetown University Medical Center, Washington, D.C.

FRED ROSNER, M.D., F.A.C.P.   Professor of Medicine, Mount Sinai School of Medicine; Director, Department of Medicine, Mount Sinai Services, Queens Hospital Center, Jamaica, New York

AVRAHAM STEINBERG, M.D.   Professor of Pediatrics, Sha'are Zadek Medical Center, Jerusalem, Israel

RABBI MOSHE TENDLER, PH.D.   Professor of Biology, Yeshiva University, New York, New York

DAVID C. THOMASMA, PH.D.   The Father Michael I. English, S.J., Professor of Medical Ethics; Director, Medical Humanities, Loyola University Chicago Stritch School of Medicine, Maywood, Illinois

Issues in Biomedical Ethics: Comparison of Jewish and Christian Perspectives

Alan I. Faden, M.D.

The origins of this book derive in large part from a conference entitled "Jewish Biomedical Ethics: Comparison with Christian and Secular Perspectives," which was conjointly sponsored by Georgetown University Medical Center and Aish Hatorah and held at Georgetown University in April 1996. The papers presented here reflect an important subset of themes from that conference and deal primarily with issues related to life and death, to suffering, and to healing. A variety of ethical problems are addressed within the context of these broad categories including active and passive euthanasia, abortion, assisted reproduction, genetic screening, and health care delivery, among others.

The book is divided into four sections. In section one, Tom Beauchamp reviews the works of Baruch Spinoza, who has been called "the greatest of the Jewish philosophers" and possibly also "the greatest of the Jewish theologians." Beauchamp reviews both Spinoza's metaphysics and his ethics. He contrasts Spinoza's perspectives on imagination and philosophy. The former was linked to theology and to faith, whereas the latter was associated with truth and reason. Beauchamp shows how Spinoza's ethics are based on a metaphysical system and compares Spinoza's distinctions between reason and faith with those of several contemporary writers. Although Spinoza respected the tradition of Jewish ethics, which is based upon classical texts and commentaries, he viewed such ethics as religious or theological as opposed to philosophical. For Spinoza, such traditions were "seriously deficient" because an understanding of ethics requires one to "transcend a specific tradition and become a philosopher."

In section two, issues relating to life and death are described from Jewish and Catholic/Christian perspectives. Baruch Brody, Ron Green, and Shimon Glick provide varied Jewish perspectives on issues relating to sanctity of life and life/death decision making. Although it is widely held that the Jewish belief in the sanctity of life implies a commitment to preserve life at all costs, each of these authors underscores the fact that the Jewish perspective is a highly nuanced one, which takes into account other values. Brody terms classical Jewish ethics a "form of pluralistic casuistry" in that it includes commitment to a variety of values, where the precedence of one value over another may vary in individual cases. In other words, there is no strict hierarchical ordering of values that is universally applied.

To underscore this point, Brody addresses two major issues: the withdrawal of life support for a dying patient and the costs of keeping a patient alive. He cites both classical texts and rabbinic commentary in arguing that under certain conditions it is permitted to remove "that which prevents the death." The assumption is that the life being prolonged cannot be saved and that the patient is suffering. When a patient is in a state termed "*goses*" or "in throes of death," it is prohibited for one to do something that prevents death. Brody argues that classical writings refer, in this case, to illness as well as imminent death; thus, withdrawal of life support under these circumstances may be consistent with the obligation not to prevent death, particularly in the presence of what he terms "unredeemed suffering." He further argues that the value to prolong human life has other limitations and may be in conflict with other values, such as eliminating suffering or limiting excessive costs to keep such a patient alive.

Green refers to Jewish religious law (*halakhah*) in discussing sanctity-of-life versus quality-of-life considerations and emphasizes the writing of Rabbi Bleich in this regard. Although the Jewish tradition supports a strong sanctity-of-life perspective, Green argues for a "more nuanced and complex view" in which other values, such as minimizing suffering, are also important considerations. He cites passages from the Talmud and the Bible claiming support for a less strict sanctity-of-life perspective in relation to the fetus than the position supported by most Orthodox Jewish bioethicists. Regarding end-of-life decisions, Green argues against the position that the quality of life should *not* be a consideration and cites both classical writings, as well as contemporary rabbinic authorities, to argue for a more nuanced perspective in which death may be considered preferable to life that is marked by "extreme physical or psychological suffering."

Glick refers to the "mythology of the infinite value of human life" and also argues for a less rigid perspective regarding the sanctity-of-life issues. Although life according to the Jewish perspective represents a divine gift that has great intrinsic value, there are circumstances under which a life may be sacrificed in support of other values, such as not violating the three cardinal sins. Glick also points out that the Torah supports the concepts of capital punishment and wars under certain prescribed conditions. Consistent with this nuanced perspective, Glick contrasts active and passive euthanasia. Although the Jewish tradition indicates a clear opposition to the active purposeful taking of a human life, Glick argues that the *halakhah* distinguishes between acts of omission and those of commission. In this regard, however, acts of omission of treatment should be for the purpose of avoiding suffering and eliminating "barriers to the natural process of death." Moreover, although under Jewish tradition it is required that an individual seek and follow medical advice for major illness, especially if there is potential risk to life, Glick argues that a patient may refuse treatment that is not life saving, particularly if it only serves to prolong the death process. He emphasizes that the treatment must be sufficient to relieve suffering, even when such treatment may shorten life. Although Glick distinguishes withdrawal therapy from withholding of therapy, he underscores the traditional view that the withdrawal of therapy is not permitted when it directly results in death.

Thomasma contrasts the Jewish and Christian perspectives regarding the sanctity-of-human-life doctrine. He traces the primary origins of the concept of the sanctity of human life within the Jewish tradition to what he terms "its salvation history," and secondarily to the biblical account of creation. Thomasma notes that the attitudes of the early church to the concept of sanctity of life were affected by the nature of certain of their converts, which included military personnel. Later, when Christianity became the official religion of the Roman Empire, it was forced to accommodate to the needs of a secular society, which included acceptance of certain forms of killing under specified conditions such as a "just war." Thomasma reviews the sanctity-of-life doctrine within the context of contemporary bioethics and describes a wide diversity of perspectives that he categorizes as "idealism," "consistent ethic of life," "respect for human life," "value of human life," "preservation of life," "antivitalism," "rationalism," and "pluralism." He concludes by presenting what he terms a "reconstruction," arguing that based upon the "collective experience of Western civilizations, human life must be intrinsically valued." Thus, for him the doctrine of the sanctity of human life becomes what he terms an "experiential *a priori.*"

The third section of the book addresses the "meaning of suffering" from Judaic and Christian perspectives. Steinberg reviews the concept of suffering in Jewish writings and underscores the point that no human is without suffering. The issue of whether suffering occurs without sin is more controversial, with classical writing both supporting and refuting this possibility. Steinberg reviews various biblical writings that attribute different explanations for sufferings: as punishment/atonement for sin; for penitence; in bringing man closer to God; to assist in bringing a person to the world to come; and, as trials that have a teaching goal. He references classical writings in suggesting that suffering is viewed as "an unwanted curse, even if it has a purpose." Nonetheless, suffering should be a learning process and lead to repentance. Steinberg contrasts the Judaic attitude toward suffering with those from other religious and philosophical writings. In contrast to Christian perspective, Steinberg indicates that the Judaic view accepts that while pain might be a punishment for sins, it does not accept the concept of original sin and does not regard suffering as a virtue or a sign of grace. Thus, even if the suffering has a purpose, one should aim to prevent and to treat it. Self-imposed suffering is forbidden.

Keenan reviews the religious response to suffering in comparing early Roman perspective, the Hebrew Bible, and the Christian tradition. He uses the work of Schillebeeckx to address Christian attitudes towards suffering, as well as misconceptions about "merited suffering" and "redemptive suffering." He supports the view of Schillebeeckx that it is a false impression of Christianity that suffering reflects an "expression of a loving God's will." He criticizes what he terms "the Christian insistence on interpreting in the face of suffering," arguing that it should be "challenged by the Jewish insistence on listening." He emphasizes the need to listen to the sufferer and emphasizes the importance of this issue for delivery of health care services. He underscores the need to allow the sufferer to communicate and to hear his or her own voice.

The fourth section deals with issues related to healing. Rosner describes the Jewish perspective, noting that the physician has a "divine license" to practice and is obligated to treat the sick person. Moreover, humans do not have "title" over their own lives or bodies and have an obligation to take care of their health. Rosner emphasizes that Judaism does not support the taking of human life except under a few prescribed conditions, such as punishment for certain capital crimes or for self-defense. It is not permitted for an individual to sacrifice his or her life to save another human life or even multiple human lives. He traces the biblical origins of the physician's imperative to heal and notes that the Bible indicates that it is an obligation. He reviews the extent of this obligation to heal where there is potential risk to the physician, such as occurs with various infectious diseases. Rosner concludes by stressing the role of the physician in cases of terminal illness, noting the prohibitions against doing that which hastens death. He reviews the types of care required for the terminally ill, including both routine care as well as the use of "potentially hazardous therapy."

Tendler reviews the Judaic and biblical perspectives regarding the applications of biomedical science, primarily relating to issues at the beginning of life, infertility, abortion, assisted reproduction, and genetic screening. He argues that the biblical duty to heal can be applied to infertility, if this is viewed as an illness. Tendler reviews the ethical concerns relating to a variety of issues such as donor insemination, ovum transplants, prolonged storage of embryos, cloning, prenatal genetic screening, and screening for disease genes. He argues that genetic screening must be linked to effective genetic counseling, that the delineation of susceptibility genes for diseases creates problems with regard to confidentiality and stigmatization, and that genetic traits cannot be used to avoid the ethical responsibility for action.

Pellegrino describes the Catholic Christian perspective regarding the imperative to heal. He indicates its derivation from the Gospels, but observes that many of its roots come from the Jewish Bible. Pellegrino notes that beginning with the acts of Jesus as a healer, healing has been an integral part of Christianity from its inception. Human life is considered a gift and it "imposes a duty of stewardship," consistent with the Jewish perspective. From this concept it follows that there is an obligation for the sick to seek treatment; however, in individual cases, this responsibility may be modified by weighing the relative costs (physical, emotional, fiscal, social) versus benefits. Pellegrino emphasizes that in the Christian tradition, spiritual healing and providing hope are important components of the overall healing process. Moreover, respect for the human person and the preservation of the dignity of the person are critical to the concept of Christian healing. From this conceptualization, suicide and euthanasia cannot be condoned.

Pellegrino discusses the implications of the Catholic Christian perspective on healing for the contemporary health professional. He emphasizes that the relationship between the health care provider and the patient cannot be contractual and should not be profit-driven; rather, this relationship should be one of a covenant, one of "promise and trust." In the same spirit, healing should be viewed as a vocation rather than an occupation. In relating the Christian perspective of healing to principles of biomedical ethics, Pellegrino notes that beneficence is a more important principle than nonmaleficence; thus, the principle of autonomy should emphasize respect for the person and dignity, and justice should be viewed as "charitable justice."

From this perspective, essential medical services should be universally accessible and equitably distributed, independent of monetary issues. In keeping with the concept of reducing suffering, health care providers should develop greater effectiveness with regard to palliative care and relief of pain. In part, this process requires "listening" to understand the causes of suffering in the individual patient.

In his paper, Cassidy summarizes the Roman Catholic teaching on the "seamless garment of life" developed by the late Cardinal Bernardin. This teaching is based in respect for life in all its manifestations from conception to death. It precludes not only abortion, euthanasia, and assisted suicide, but capital punishment and killing except in self-defense or in wars that satisfy the criteria of a just war. Father Cassidy's explication of the Catholic respect for life is grounded in the Old Testament doctrine of the *Imago Dei*, but also in the embryological development of the human conceptus.

In comparing these bioethical issues from Jewish and Christian perspectives, it is important to underscore several points. First, although the authors present largely consistent views within each tradition, these perspectives may not reflect the full diversity of positions within either the Jewish or Christian traditions. Thus, contributors addressing Jewish bioethics largely reflect an orthodox perspective, with an emphasis on Jewish religious law (*halakhah*). Similarly, the Christian "perspective" reflects a Catholic Christian viewpoint. Nonetheless, many of the authors describe competing underlying ethical values and review what appear at times to be conflicting sources in examining these issues. Second, in reviewing this Jewish-Catholic Christian dialogue, it is apparent that although the two traditions present remarkably compatible positions on many of the issues (after all, the roots of Christianity derive from the Jewish Bible), it is also evident that these similar perspectives often reflect a distinctly different conceptual basis. For example, the Jewish viewpoints are based upon Old Testament sources and emphasize Jewish law. In contrast, Christian perspectives also emphasize New Testament sources and appeal to faith. These distinctions are most clearly articulated in the sections relating to euthanasia and to healing.

It is our hope that the Jewish/Christian dialogue, initiated with the 1996 conference and as reflected with this book, will continue in the future. In this regard, it is perhaps noteworthy that the impetus for this book came from the conference presenters rather than the conference organizers.

Ethics as Philosophy

Spinoza and Judaism

Tom L. Beauchamp, Ph.D.

Baruch (or Benedict) Spinoza (b. Amsterdam, 24 November 1632; d. 21 February 1677) was among the most important philosophers in early modern Europe and has often been called the greatest of the Jewish philosophers—possibly also the greatest of the Jewish theologians. The oddity of this ranking of Spinoza, as we will have a chance to discuss, is that his greatest book is titled *Ethics*, yet he has had little impact on what is ordinarily thought of as Jewish ethics. But before we get to these peculiarities, I will mention something about Spinoza's life and philosophy.

Spinoza came from a family of Portuguese and Spanish Jews who fled to Holland in order to escape the Spanish Inquisition. He was born in 1632, the same year as the second condemnation of Galileo before the Roman Inquisition (1616, 1632). Only a few years previously, Giordano Bruno had been tried by the Inquisition for his scientific and philosophical beliefs and burned at the stake in 1600. This was a difficult period, with great fears in Spinoza's family that the Inquisition would spread. Spinoza was never able to escape the troubled religious times, and his philosophical views ultimately satisfied not a single one of the troubled parties.

Spinoza's father was a religious Jew and had become a prominent member of the synagogue in Amsterdam. Clearly gifted from an early age, Spinoza was educated at the Jewish Academy, where he was taught Hebrew, the Bible, the Talmud, and the Kabbalah, as well as medieval Jewish philosophy and theology, studying figures such as Maimonides and Gersonides. Still young, however, Spinoza began to doubt much of the theology he had been taught and started to develop his own system. He came under suspicion by the Jewish theologians, and consequently he held back from full participation in the synagogue.

He soon read Descartes, who shaped much of his terminology and thinking. After 1651 (the year Hobbes published the *Leviathan*) Spinoza read the Stoics, Renaissance Neoplatonists, Calvinist Scholastics, Latin classics, and mathematics. One of the great ironies is that Spinoza, even as a Jew, loved the Scholastics and appears to have taken more from them than any modern philosopher.

These diverse influences drove Spinoza still farther away from the conventional Jewish beliefs in which he had been trained. In 1656, at age 24, he was expelled from the synagogue. The Protestant clergy also feared him, and for a period he was forced to leave Amsterdam. Eventually he moved to the Hague where he lived for the rest of his life. He vigorously but vainly sought to seclude himself in an environment of tranquillity and to avoid any invitations that would compromise his freedom of thought and speech. So covetous was Spinoza of his intellectual freedom that he turned down the offer of a chair in philosophy at Heidelberg—on grounds that pressures might be brought on him to hold certain views. By now he was internationally famous and many scholars sought him out at his home.

Spinoza published only two books in his lifetime. The first was on Descartes' philosophy. The second, titled *Theologico-Political Treatise* (1660), was regarded at the time as quintessentially atheistic and was published anonymously. [1] Spinoza's experience with the *Theologico-Political Treatise* led him to think that his work on ethics would be a bombshell. He therefore carefully guarded access to his *Ethics*, revising it repeatedly, but never publishing it.

INTELLECT (REASON) AND IMAGINATION

In his *Ethics* Spinoza attempted to construct a geometrically ordered system of abstract, intuitively certain propositions and logically necessary deductions. Reason, and no other faculty, was the sole means to the construction of such a system.

In order to construct a philosophical system, Spinoza thought, one must totally abandon the sense-derived images of the faculty of imagination in favor of the common notions or adequate ideas of the intellect. In the *Ethics* he attempted to practice what he proclaimed by passing from that which is imagistic in character to adequate ideas deduced from clear and distinct ideas that are their own standard of truth.

Spinoza thought that we are sometimes fooled because images seem more vivid and understandable than abstract truths. It is not too much to say that his whole philosophy represents a progressive movement away from the imagination toward a total reliance on reason, and as we will see, this vision affected in the deepest possible way how he viewed both philosophy and religious belief. The list below shows how deeply Spinoza's fundamental bifurcation between imagination and intellect runs.

IMAGINATION contrasts with *INTELLECT (REASON)*

associated with	*associated with*
Inadequate ideas	Adequate ideas
Pictures (images)	Clear and distinct ideas
Images externally caused	Ideas internally concatenated
Falsity, fictions	Truth
Passive reception	Active formulation
Theology	Philosophy
Faith	Reason
Images of finite objects	Idea of infinity
Anthropomorphism	Idea of God

MATHEMATICAL IDEAL

Spinoza looked for knowledge of the objective rational order of things, which he took to be the opposite of the imagined order. Reason finds objective truth and arranges it in perfect order—a logical order. Spinoza wanted a complete system of universal truths that was eternal and necessary. As was typical of rationalist philosophers with whom he is commonly associated, he based the necessary relations on a knowledge of causal necessity. Spinoza, we might say, wanted to understand the causal order of the universe as a unified system because that universe is God's universe; indeed, the universe is God in this metaphysics.

ETHICAL ORIENTATION

But Spinoza's work is not merely a metaphysics; it is an ethics based on a metaphysical system. Spinoza thought enough of this interconnection to give the title *Ethics* to his work: [2] his system of thought is intended not only to culminate in a treatise on ethics, but to construct and to understand that the system is in itself the proper (ethical) way of life. In this sense, the book not only specifies what you should do, but actually does it.

The *Ethics* is Spinoza's attempt to overcome the temptations of fame, riches, and sensuality—any kind of worldly corrupting influence—in favor of true understanding and a worthwhile goal in life—to gain freedom, to achieve perfection, and even to possess immortality in the only meaningful sense of that term. The overall goal was to provide a program for the perfection of human nature. [3]

Spinoza thought that just as a geometrical science can be constructed on the basis of self-evident postulates, so a science of reality and ethics can be constructed. For example, by definition of "substance" (and here Spinoza follows Descartes), it is "what is in itself and conceived through itself." [4] If God is the substance, as religious traditions suggest, then everything will depend strictly on God and there will be no substance other than God.

Spinoza thought that properly constructed definitions show insight into the nature of things: definitions are definitions of something, and reason is capable of constructing definitions that adequately capture that of which they are definitions. This point must be grasped if Spinoza's method is to be understood. In mathematical or formal sciences, definitions and axioms function as grounds from which other propositions are logically deduced. These relations are not usually thought to be *causal* relations, because temporal relations and empirical conditions are not logical considerations. Spinoza, however, thought of the two sorts of relations—logical and causal—as close, if not identical. A cause, then, is a reason or ground for an effect; no important distinction was thought by Spinoza to exist between logical relations (which are conceptual) and causal relations (which are empirical).

It is not hard to understand why Spinoza thought there was no important difference. In both cases, so he believed, the relation (of entailment) is a necessary one. Given the cause, the effect must follow; just as given a proposition, that which it entails must follow. [5] Spinoza regarded the universe as a causal chain in which each link of the chain is necessarily connected to another link, much as conclusions are logically linked to the premises from which they are deduced (a concatenation or connection in each case). A basic axiom in Spinoza's thought is the strict correlation between thought and reality: the order and connection of ideas is identical to the order and connection of things. As he develops this correlation, a universal determinism is the outcome. If one grasped the whole system of reality, one would grasp all the necessary causal relations—just as in geometry, if one grasped the whole system of geometry, one would grasp all the necessary logical relations.

It is easy to misunderstand this point. Just as Euclid was not interested in particular triangles or relations or other geometrical objects, so Spinoza is not interested in particular causal items or relations. He is like a scientist in that he is interested in general causal relations—i.e., general causal laws. His ambition is to see the general order of things as an interrelated system. Any particular thing is to be understood only by subsumption under these laws.

Moreover, Spinoza thought, laws are omnitemporal and omnispatial in character. So to grasp the system of laws is to grasp eternal relations—just as in mathematics we deal with eternal, not temporal, items. Hence, to do metaphysics is to grasp things—or, better, laws—*sub specie aeternitatis* ("under a species of eternity"). [6] His metaphysics is this system of laws, and his ethics is based on it.

THE ROLE OF THE IMAGINATION: FALSITY AND FICTIONS

I return now to Spinoza's philosophy of the imagination. The function of the imagination is to represent objects as if they were present. Spinoza believed the objects and events that we meet in experience are generally grasped only through rather faulty pictures that represent the objects in an inadequate manner:

> For an imagination is an idea which indicates the present constitution of the human Body more than the nature of an external body—not distinctly, of course, but confusedly. This is how it happens that the Mind is said to err. [7]

REASON

The confused ideas of the imagination (images) are inadequate ideas because they reflect only the momentary and unrelated condition of the body as it is affected by external objects. Reason or understanding (intellect) rescues us from the inadequacy of images. Spinoza's discussion of God in Part 1 of the *Ethics* is conducted in precisely this manner. God is understood only insofar as the mind is purged of images (such as anthropomorphic pictures) and enabled thereby to grasp God's essence through clearly defined definitions and axioms that are self-evident or necessary.

Spinoza used the term "intuitive knowledge" to refer to a detailed, comprehensive grasp of the entire system or nexus of causal connectedness, including how everything that exists is necessarily grounded (causally or logically) in the ultimate ground of nature—God. [8]

GOD

In some philosophies the ultimate factor in the system of thought is some sort of substance, while in others it is God. For Spinoza, whether it is God or substance or nature is really an unimportant semantical question. God, substance, and nature are (extensionally) identical, even though there may be an (intensional) difference in the way they are defined. [9]

Spinoza seems to say that God, his nature, his power, and the laws of his nature, and his attributes are equivalent; and I think we should emphasize laws of nature. Here is what Spinoza has to say in the *Ethics*: [10]

> [N]ature is always the same, and its virtue and power of acting are everywhere one and the same, i.e., the laws and rules of nature, according to which all things happen, and change from one form to another, are always and everywhere the same. So the way of understanding the nature of anything, of whatever kind, must also be the same, *viz.* through the universal laws and rules of nature.

FREEDOM AND DETERMINISM

Parts 4 and 5 (some of 3) of the *Ethics* concentrate on many topics surrounding the problem of freedom and determinism that emanates from this account of universal law. Spinoza, of course, did not exempt human beings from the rigorous system of causes in nature that he constructed. There is no faculty of free will, and there is no indeterminism in the universe. Even so, Spinoza thought a meaning can be given to human freedom. His strategy was to acknowledge that persons are often the slaves of powerful passions but that they can be made free by freeing themselves from these passions. Slaves and free persons are not different because one is determined and the other not determined. They are different in that a slave is subject to a master. Spinoza's theory of freedom is a theory concerning how one can remove oneself from slavery to the passions and the imagination (closely associated with the passions for Spinoza) through adequate ideas. To the extent that the mind is active in understanding rather than passive, bondage is overcome. [11]

Spinoza's idea seems to be that once a person rationally understands that the universe is governed by necessity (a system of laws), the person will be differently affected by the events apprehended and can act in accordance with this knowledge, making the person joyous, virtuous, and free. For example, once a person experiencing greed understands that fact and also understands how all persons are (necessarily) determined, the person will come to understand why others, oneself included, might be greedy. In understanding the causes of greed, one is able to surmount being greedy as well as to surmount feeling ill towards others who are greedy. The person shall cease then to be greedy or to wish others ill. The Jewish belief is similar; understanding enables the sick to overcome the effects of the sickness and to understand the sickness of others. It enables an appropriate response.

ETHICS

When Spinoza discussed the highest state to which persons can aspire, he recommended a state of mental tranquillity or rest in which God is accepted as absolutely good. Persons should love God without any expectation of love or benefit in return. The chief contribution philosophy can make to moral practice is to show how such a life is possible, given all the distractions in life and the diverting power of the imagination. In the end, love of God is the final aim of every wise person's life. In Part 5 of his *Ethics*, Spinoza gave the final stage of human freedom, which involves transforming all passion into action in the form of an "intellectual love of God." [12] Here human nature is perfected, and we intuit our unity and fellowship with God. This stage both liberates and confers immortality. In this way, philosophy substitutes for religiously derived moral ideals of life. Spinoza thus has a model vision of the way you ought to live your life, and obviously it is more philosophically than theologically oriented.

THE THEOLOGICO-POLITICAL TREATISE

I turn, finally, to Spinoza's views about religion, ethics, and philosophy as they were pursued in his early work. This work was fiercely denounced by orthodox religionists of all faiths and was legally banned in many countries. In the Preface to the *Theologico-Political Treatise*, Spinoza unambiguously stated his position on the relation of philosophy to theology (Jewish and Christian): "The Bible leaves reason absolutely free [and] . . . has nothing in common with philosophy. . . . Revelation and Philosophy stand on totally different footings." [13] The aim of philosophy is truth; the goal of religion and theology is obedience. Hence the two can never conflict if they are kept separate and functioning in their proper domains.

Spinoza's diligent research into Scripture led him to the conclusion that the intention of the persons whose prophecies and writings fill the Bible was not philosophical or scientific or historical, but moral and religious. Their words were aimed at instilling obedience, not knowledge, in those followers who heard their proclamations. They performed this task not by adequate ideas and rational proofs, but by adapting their exhortations to ideas of the imagination (also the source for perceiving revelations) that were acceptable and easily understood by their listeners and readers. Spinoza argued that the

Scriptures are for the masses who do not understand clearly and distinctly. This gives room for theologians, who tend to embellish and exaggerate scriptural claims.

In what some will no doubt judge a grossly condescending attitude, Spinoza held that theologians and the masses of religious believers uncritically accept the Scriptures because the accounts contained therein can "most powerfully dispose their mind [imagination] to obedience and devotion." [14] Not intellectual reasons but imaginative delight in the stories related by Scripture determines acceptance; and the demand that Scripture itself makes is not intellectual assent but absolute obedience and devotion.

Spinoza was able to distinguish philosophical knowledge from revelation as given in Scripture largely because of the separate functions of intellect and imagination. He regarded the prophets as men peculiarly gifted with strong, "unusually vivid imaginations," though not with "unusually perfect minds" for "abstract reasoning" by the intellect. [15] The prophets obtain revelations through special imaginative insights, though their prophetic messages are inevitably colored by individual temperament, previous beliefs, education, historical situation, etc. Furthermore, the prophet must appeal to the imagination of his hearers in order to communicate his vision.

Spinoza said that no real knowledge of "natural and spiritual phenomena" is gained by the prophet. In fact "prophecy never rendered the prophet wiser than he was before," and his imagination does not "involve any certainty of truth." [16] The peculiar power of imagining that prophets possess is simply a gift as rare as the ability of "composing poetry *extempore*." [17]

The prophets' images also function to guide human conduct. The object and substance of revelations are admonitions to lead the good and true life. Prophets proclaim attributes of God that persons are able to imitate. They seek to impress on the imagination of their hearers "that God is supremely just, and supremely merciful—in other words, the one perfect pattern of the true life." [18] This is why religion is popular and why it is admired in a culture: It delivers, with divine authority, how you should live your life, which is as a form of obedience to God; and obedience to God is carried out through the love of neighbors.

Theological ethics is for Spinoza the discipline that explains the images of God that depict him as an exemplar or paradigm of justice and charity for all human conduct. It is therefore to be completely separated from philosophy. For Spinoza, philosophy and theology are "as wide apart as the poles." [19] "Imagination and intellect, faith and reason—these polarities stand forever separate, each functioning for a different purpose." [20]

Spinoza claimed that Scripture nowhere gives either a definition of God or a knowledge of God's attributes other than those of justice and mercy. Theologians who would explain miracles as unique, theistic, supernatural suspensions of these laws only display their ignorance of philosophy and of Scripture's true intent. The task of theology is to explain correctly and faithfully what Scripture says, not to reinforce and interpret it with philosophical reasons.

EVALUATION AND CONCLUSION

However overstated and even pretentious Spinoza's views may seem to us today, his account is not at all implausible, especially if one makes a sharp distinction between reason and faith, as many theologians and philosophers have done. Moreover, Spinoza's views are not without their contemporary counterparts. For example, R. B. Braithwaite's monograph *An Empiricist's View of the Nature of Religious Belief* [21] is a sustained argument to the conclusion that religious assertions are not matters of truth or falsity, because they are at bottom religious and moral prescriptions and proscriptions. (For Braithwaite it is not even necessary that religious stories be believed to be true by believers.) Religious statements thus express a commitment to a general way of life, not to a body of truths. Braithwaite finds the difference between particular religious traditions in the different stories, myths, and parables uniquely associated with those particular traditional ways of life.

If one turns away from philosophical accounts of religion to the work of contemporary theologians, and in particular to theological ethics, one can find what strikes me as substantially similar accounts. Stanley Hauerwas, for example, has argued that a religious community (its "form and substance") is shaped by narrative and by commitment to the authority of Scripture. He holds that moral communities make us what we are, and moral communities are constituted by a narrative tradition. In his view, a moral outlook is defensible only within such a tradition, and the great mistake of modern philosophical ethics has been to suppose that there could be a nonnarrative, tradition-free theory of either religion or normative ethics. [22]

Hauerwas and Spinoza are wholly at odds on the place of philosophy, but note their agreements about religion. They both see Scripture and religious tradition as instilling a moral way of life and a form of religious obedience. This is accomplished by nonphilosophical means, because it is rooted in stories that stand as exemplars of conduct. Both see theology's proper task as that of the faithful explanation of what Scripture says, and they see a philosophical apologetics as a perversion of the role of the theologian.

Now, I have said nothing at all about Jewish ethics in the course of this lecture. Jewish ethics is derived from classical Jewish texts and the reflections of scholars about the teachings in those texts—stretching from the biblical, talmudic, medieval, to modern periods. It is just these sources that Spinoza thought of as religious and theological rather than philosophical. While he deeply respected and drew from these traditions, especially biblical accounts of the prophets, the great Jewish mystics, and the Jewish idea of universal law applicable to everyone, there is an important sense in which all parts of this tradition are, from his perspective, seriously deficient. To really understand ethics and the doctrine of God, a person must transcend a specific tradition and become a philosopher.

NOTES

1. Benedict de Spinoza, *Theologico-Political Treatise*, trans. R. Elwes in *The Chief Works of Benedict de Spinoza*, vol. 1 (New York: Dover Books, 1951).
2. Benedict de Spinoza, *Ethics* in *The Collected Works of Spinoza*, vol. 1, ed. and trans. Edwin Curley (Princeton: Princeton University Press, 1985; second printing, with corrections, 1988).
3. These demonstrations are entirely deductive from intuitively certain premises, as in geometry; and each proof of a proposition ends with the inscription "Q.E.D.," and with corollaries and scholia. Spinoza uses definitions, axioms, and postulates to move to propositions, demonstrations, corollaries, scholia, and lemmata.
4. Benedict de Spinoza, *Ethics*, Pt. 1, Def. 3 (p. 408).
5. To make another parallel, in a formally valid argument, conclusions (which are propositions) follow logically from premises (which are propositions). The premises necessitate the conclusion. Similarly in metaphysics, Spinoza thought, in a correct statement of causal relatedness, effects follow from a cause or set of causes. The cause necessitates the effect.
6. Benedict de Spinoza, *Ethics*, Pt. 5, p.22 and schol. (p. 607).
7. Benedict de Spinoza, *Ethics*, Pt. 4, p.1, schol. (p. 547). "This proposition is understood more clearly from II–P16–C2," Spinoza reports.
8. Benedict de Spinoza, *Ethics*, Pt. 2, p.40, schol. 2, [IV]; Pt. 4, Appx. IV; Pt. 5, schol.
9. This is obvious from the very first paragraphs in the *Ethics*. See Pt. 1, Defs. 3 ("substance") and 6 ("God"). Defs. 2 ("finite") and 4 ("attribute") make it obvious that only substance can have infinite attributes.
10. Benedict de Spinoza, *Ethics*, Pt. 3, Preface.
11. Benedict de Spinoza, *Ethics*, Pt. 4.
12. Benedict de Spinoza, *Ethics*, Pt. 5, pp. 32–37.
13. Benedict de Spinoza, *Theologico-Political Treatise*, p. 9.
14. Benedict de Spinoza, *Theologico-Political Treatise*, p. 79.
15. Benedict de Spinoza, *Theologico-Political Treatise*, p. 27.

16. Benedict de Spinoza, *Theologico-Political Treatise*, pp. 27f.

17. Benedict de Spinoza, *Theologico-Political Treatise*, note 3 of p. 24 (printed on pp. 269f).

18. Benedict de Spinoza, *Theologico-Political Treatise*, p. 179.

19. Benedict de Spinoza, *Theologico-Political Treatise*, p. 189.

20. Benedict de Spinoza, *Theologico-Political Treatise*, pp. 42, 95f, 178–81.

21. R. B. Braithwaite, *An Empiricist's View of the Nature of Religious Belief* (Cambridge: Cambridge University Press, 1955).

22. Stanley Hauerwas, *A Community of Character: Toward a Constructive Christian Social Ethic* (Notre Dame, Ind.: University of Notre Dame Press, 1981), pp. 95–97.

SECTION TWO

The Sanctity of Human Life

Jewish Reflections on Life and Death Decision Making

BARUCH A. BRODY, PH.D.

It is widely believed that the classical Jewish view on life and death decision making is based on a belief in the sanctity of human life and is committed to the preservation of that life at any cost. [1] It is understandable why this is believed; classical Judaism certainly ascribes great value to human life and its preservation. Nevertheless, this belief is mistaken. I shall in this paper present some of the evidence that the classical Jewish view is a far more nuanced view, one that accommodates the significance of other values including the recognition that death is sometimes a benefit, that pain and suffering must be minimized, and that excessive social costs of preserving life cannot be sustained. [2]

That the classical Jewish view is more nuanced should not come as a surprise. Sanctity-of-life views are committed to the belief that one value always takes precedence over all other values. Classical Jewish ethics is not structured in that way. It is committed to the legitimacy of a wide variety of values, and it recognizes that which value takes precedence varies from one case to the other. In this way, classical Jewish ethics is a form of pluralistic casuistry. [3] This explains why its main texts (including the Talmud and its commentaries, the codes and their commentaries, and the responsa literature) are focused on a consideration of an ever-expanding number of cases, with no attempt made to resolve them by appeal to a few fundamental principles or to some hierarchical structure of values.

This paper will contain two major sections. The first will deal with issues related to the withdrawal of life support because the patient is dying and no longer wishes to suffer. The second will deal with issues related to the cost of keeping patients alive. In both cases, we will see the interplay of multiple values as the tradition attempts to deal with these problems in a nuanced fashion.

THE WITHDRAWAL OF LIFE SUPPORT

The classic texts permitting the withdrawal of that which is keeping a patient alive are a series of comments by R. Moshe Isserles (the sixteenth century author of definitive glosses on the major codes). Drawing upon earlier sources, Isserles says:

> It is prohibited to cause someone to die quicker, as in the case of someone who has been a *goses* for a long time ... But if there is something that causes a delay in the death ... it is permitted to remove it, for that is not an act, but the taking away of that which prevents the death. [4]

Several of the classical commentators on Isserles's glosses add as the reason for permitting the removal of that which prevents the death that it is wrong for it to be there because it causes unjustified pain and suffering. This line of thought led the revered R. Moshe Feinstein, the leading twentieth century American author of responsa literature, to conclude:

> It seems to me that since there is in this medical care only the capacity to extend his life a short time, if this short time that he will live with this medical help is with a lot of pain, it is prohibited ... Probably this is the reason that it is permissible to take away that which prevents the death. [5]

There are a number of crucial points that need to be made about these texts to insure that their relevance to the contemporary bioethical discussion is fully appreciated.

First, there is the clear recognition that the person's continued life may be bad for that person. The continued existence of the terminally ill is often filled with unredeemed pain and suffering. This is particularly true of those whose dying has been a lengthy process. This recognition led Nissim of Gerondi, the classic fourteenth century commentator, to conclude (drawing on the talmudic story relating to the death of Judah the Prince, the author of the Mishna) that "there are times that one needs to pray about the sick person that he should die since he is in a great deal of pain because of his illness and he cannot live." [6]

Second, this recognition leads to the conclusion that it is permitted to both withhold and withdraw that which prevents the patient from dying. The withdrawal is permitted as the consequence of the permissibility of not providing it to begin with. In many of the texts, a concern is expressed that the withdrawal may, in some cases, cause the death of the patient by moving the patient's body, and a caution on that point is expressed with varying degrees of severity. [7] Fortunately, in the contemporary setting, those interventions which most often prevent the patient from dying (e.g., pressors, respiratory support) can be withdrawn without even touching the patient's body.

Third, the patients in question are those who are dying. Technically, they are in the state called *goses*. There are contemporary commentators, most notably J. David Bleich, [8] who have insisted that this is the state of the patient in the throes of death who will die in the next three days regardless of the best care provided. This is not the place to examine the texts cited by them to prove this assertion. It suffices for our purposes to note that the text of Isserles quoted above directly proves the opposite, since Isserles talks of someone who has been a *goses* for a long time. [9] We are dealing with those who are terminally ill and who are suffering, but not necessarily in the throes of death.

Fourth, the texts in question do not talk merely about the permissibility of withholding/withdrawing that which impedes the patient from dying. They talk about the prohibition of prolonging life when it cannot be saved and when the patient is suffering. Another gloss of Isserles [10] makes this clear: "It is certainly prohibited to do something that will cause him not to die." The importance of this point cannot be overemphasized. The discussion has for too long centered on the *permissibility* of foregoing life support. It is time to focus it on the *prohibition* to continue life support in certain cases. Particularly in talking to families who insist that "everything be done," it has become my practice to challenge them with the question as to why we are permitted to cause extra suffering to dying patients if we cannot save them. The relevance of this point to the current discussion about futile interventions is obvious. The recent Houston protocol [11] that allows physicians to refuse to pointlessly prolong the suffering of dying patients is very compatible with this classical Judaic perspective.

Fifth, the texts in question emphasize the centrality of pain and suffering in this setting. As the hospice movement regularly reminds us, proper pain control leads to fewer requests to die. This seems correct, but there are those who have misunderstood this point. Bleich, in a recent essay, [12] has questioned the applicability of this whole set of classical texts on the grounds that adequate pain support is now available to the terminally ill. He quotes in this connection Dr. Porter Storey who has written about his success in managing the pain of the dying. Dr. Storey, both a colleague and a friend, is indeed remarkably successful in this effort. But he has been so in his role of medical director of a hospice, and a central component of the palliation he can provide his patients is that he does not provide interventions that prevent them from dying and that needlessly prolong the suffering that would then become harder and harder to control. It is ironical that his experience is used in arguing for the provision of just these interventions in direct contradiction to the hospice philosophy, and he has authorized me to say that it should not be used in supporting this contradictory approach.

Finally, the texts quoted until now have little to say about the role of patient autonomy. This is not surprising, since that theme is not as central in classical Jewish ethics as it is in contemporary American bioethics. Nevertheless, there are other texts which introduce it to some degree as well. This is not surprising, since the meaning of pain will differ from one individual to another. One of the most interesting of these texts is a responsum from R. Shlomo Zalman Auerbach, the recently deceased leading Israeli religious authority. In it, he says:

> Probably, however, if the sick person is suffering a lot of physical pain, or even if he is in great psychological pain, I believe that we are obliged to give him food and oxygen against his wishes, but we can withhold treatment that causes pain if he requests it. But if he is pious and will not become despondent, it is desirable to explain to him that one moment of repentance in this world is more valuable than all of the world to come. [13]

Several points should be noted about this text: (a) food and oxygen are placed in a separate category, for unspecified reasons; (b) the individual makes the decision about the life support in light of the pain; (c) there is continued religious value in staying alive, the possibility of using that time for religious purposes, but only if one is cognitively intact; (d) the pain can be psychological as well as physical. This observation is particularly important when reflecting on dying patients in the late stages of degenerative neuromuscular diseases, who experience great psychological frustration and resulting distress rather than physical pain.

What has emerged from a careful reading of these texts is obviously not a sanctity-of-life position. Instead, it is a nuanced balancing of many values. The prolongation of human life, as long as it does not involve unredeemed pain and suffering, is a great value. A cure or long-term control of the disease is one such redeeming value, but another is the use to which the time can be put. In the latter cases, the patient must choose. But if the pain and suffering is unredeemed, then it is wrong to use measures that prolong the dying of the patient, and if these measures are already in place, they may/must be withdrawn. Care should be taken not to directly kill the patient in that process. These principles apply to all dying patients experiencing pain and suffering, and not just to those in the throes of death.

THE COST OF LIFE SUPPORT

In all of the above-cited texts, the question of the cost of maintaining the dying patient on life support is not raised. There are, moreover, no other classical texts which directly raise that issue. That issue has only become relevant in the last few decades, where technological advances have enabled physicians to keep dying patients alive at great expense. To what extent should that cost be considered in clinical decision making? Obviously, those who believe in the sanctity or in the infinite value of human life will conclude that it should not be considered, and this conclusion has been supported in the literature on Jewish bioethics. I will now argue that there are classical texts, dealing with other issues of the saving of lives, that suggest otherwise.

In order to appreciate the relevance of these texts, it is necessary to provide some background about the classical Jewish position on the obligation to save the lives of others, even those who are strangers. The existence of this obligation, often referred to as the Good Samaritan obligation, was rejected in the common law. But classical Jewish law and ethics insisted that it did exist. It posited both a negative obligation ("Thou shall not stand idly by and allow the death of thy friend") and a positive obligation ("Return it to him") to prevent where possible the loss of life. These obligations were given great weight, and the existence of the dual obligation was interpreted as requiring both personal effort and the expenditure of one's own funds. These obligations are obviously applicable to the medical setting, but they were articulated in other contexts (e.g., saving the drowning, redeeming those who had been captured to be sold into life-threatening slavery). And it is in one of these other settings, the setting of the obligation to redeem captives, that the economic question is raised.

The classical text is a report of a rabbinic decree found in the Babylonian Talmud:

> Captives should not be redeemed for more than their value, to prevent abuses . . . The question was raised: Does this prevention of abuses relate to the burden which may be imposed upon the community or to the possibility that the activities [of the bandits] may be stimulated. Come and hear: Levi b. Darga ransomed his daughter for 13,000 denari of

gold. Said Abaye: But are you sure that he acted with the consent of the sages? Perhaps he acted against the will of the sages? [14]

Of the two interpretations, only the first interprets this decree in a way that makes it directly relevant to our concerns. Only it makes the economic burdens on the community the basis for not being obliged to save the lives of the captives by redeeming them; only on this interpretation of the rabbinic decree could it serve as a precedent for saying that excessive economic burdens free the community from the obligation to provide life-prolonging interventions. The second interpretation sees this decree as addressing the issue of allowing the current captives to die (by not redeeming them) so that more will live in the future (because more captives will not be taken). While its interpretation would make the decree relevant to other issues in medical ethics, it makes it irrelevant to our concerns. This observation needs to be supplemented by several additional observations.

First, the question of which interpretation has been adopted as definitive is a matter of some controversy. [15] A superficial reading of the major codes, without an examination of their commentators, would certainly suggest that it was the second interpretation that was adopted. A close examination of the major sixteenth through seventeenth century authors such as Bach, Shach, Maharshal, and Radbaz reveals that they explicitly or implicitly adopted the first interpretation. I see no reason therefore not to use it as a precedent for the medical setting.

Second, it is important to keep in mind that the captives, if redeemed, would usually live a regular life span, but that those dependent on expensive life support, even if maintained on that support, often would not. If the economic burden on the community is a sufficient justification for not redeeming the captives, it should *a fortiori* be a sufficient justification for not maintaining those patients on life support.

Third, this economic limitation on providing life support may be far broader than the above-discussed pain-based limitation on providing life support. This economic limitation refers only to the expense of the intervention and the burden it imposes upon the community; such a burden may be present even in patients who could live for a long time without being in pain if the support is provided. A good example of this is the case of the otherwise healthy persistent vegetative patient, who by definition suffers no pain, but whose long-term support can be very expensive and a burden on the community. If this decree provides a precedent for the medical setting, it may justify on economic grounds the provision of life-prolonging interventions to such patients.

Fourth, as the above-cited text indicates, the objection to spending so much money is that it excessively burdens the community. None of this is relevant to the question of what the individual or his/her family and friends may spend to save the individual's life. On the first interpretation, this is why Levi b. Darga could spend so much money to redeem his daughter. In the medical setting, this means that the limitation is on the public obligation to spend funds to provide life-supporting medical interventions. A second more extensive tier of medical care, supported by private funds and providing ever more expensive interventions with ever less likelihood of success, is not ruled out by this rabbinic decree. In this respect, this classical Jewish text provides a precedent for the conclusion of the President's Commission [16] that the social obligation to provide even life-prolonging interventions is not unlimited, even when additional interventions are available and are being purchased by some from private funds. People are free to spend their money as they see fit once their moral/religious obligations to others are met. It is of course a separate question as to whether this use of private funds is wise or fitting.

Fifth, the precise nature of the economic limitation on the first interpretation is very unclear. On the second interpretation, there is a standard account: do not redeem the captives for more than the usual rate, for paying more will encourage more taking of captives. But how should the limitation be understood according to the first interpretation? And what does it mean in the health care setting? I think that the following needs to be said by way of a beginning: the crucial theme is protecting the community from being excessively burdened. This theme and its correlates must structure the answer, keeping in mind that the community has other needs that it must meet from public funds and that individuals must have private funds to enable them to explore and develop their own goals. It comes then to a percentage of the community's total assets that must be devoted to life-prolonging/saving activities. This percentage may not be fixed; it may grow as the wealth of the community grows (being in this way a progressive as opposed to a proportional system). Even if it does not, so that it is a proportional system, the absolute number of dollars available for such purposes will grow as the wealth of the community grows. On the other hand, the existence of other pressing needs may limit the percentage, and the percentage will in any case purchase less life-prolonging/saving activities as the number in need of these activities grows. None of this is a complete account; crucially missing is a theory of how the base percentage must be fixed.

What has emerged from these reflections is hardly an infinite-value-of-human-life position. Instead, it is a nuanced balancing of both the value of providing life support to those whose life is threatened and the values embodied in various other communal responsibilities and individual projects. In a world of infinite resources, these values would not need to be balanced. In the real world of limited resources, they do, and classical Jewish casuistry calls for doing just that.

NOTES

1. See, for example, Ezekiel Emanuel, "A Communal Vision of Care for Incompetent Patients," *Hastings Center Report,* vol. 17, no. 5 (1987): 15–20.

2. More is presented in "A Historical Introduction to Jewish Casuistry on Suicide and Euthanasia" in Baruch Brody, ed., *Suicide and Euthanasia: Historical and Contemporary Themes* (Dordrecht: Kluwer Academic Publishers, 1989): 39–76 and in Baruch Brody, "The Economics of the Laws of Rodef," *Svara,* vol. 1, no. 1(1990): 67–69.

3. Of the sort defended in Baruch Brody, *Life and Death Decision Making* (New York: Oxford University Press, 1988).

4. Isserles on *Shulchan Aruch* Y.D. 339:1.

5. *Igrot Moshe* Y.D. II, #174.

6. R. Nissim on Alfasi, *Nedarim* 40a.

7. See the opinions cited on pp. 369–70 of vol. 4 of Abraham Steinberg's *Encyclopedia Halacit-Refuit* (Jerusalem: Machon Schlesinger, 1994).

8. Most recently in J. David Bleich, "Treatment of the Terminally Ill," *Tradition,* vol. 30, no. 3 (1996): 51–87.

9. I have long advocated this point as a disproof of Bleich's assertion. I am delighted to find this argument supported by Abraham Steinberg in footnote 130a on p. 368 of vol. 4 of his *Encyclopedia Halachit-Refuit,* (Jerusalem: Machon Schlesinger, 1994).

10. Darkei Moshe on *Tur* YD 339:1.

11. Amir Halevy and Baruch Brody, "A Multi-Institution Collaborative Policy on Medical Futility," *JAMA,* vol. 276 (August 21, 1966): 571–74. This has recently been supported by the AMA's House of Delegates.

12. J. David Bleich, "Treatment of the Terminally Ill," *Tradition,* vol. 30, no. 3 (1996): 51–87.

13. Shlomo Zalman Auerbach, "Caring for a Dying Patient" in M. Hershler, ed., *Halacha U'Refuah,* vol. 2 (Jerusalem: Regensburg Institute, 1981): 131.

14. *Gittin* 45a.

15. An excellent discussion of this and related issues about this decree is to be found in Israel Schepansky's *Hatakanot B'Yisrael,* vol. 2 (Jerusalem: Mosad Rav Kook, 1992): 51–56.

16. President's Commission, *Securing Access to Health Care* (Washington: Government Printing Office, 1983).

Jewish Teaching on the Sanctity and Quality of Life

Ronald M. Green, Ph.D.

In April 1996 in an emotionally charged White House ceremony, President Clinton vetoed a bill that would have banned almost all so-called "partial-birth" abortions. This rare procedure, usually employed during the third trimester, involves piece-by-piece removal of a fetus from its mother's womb in order to terminate the pregnancy. The procedure is characterized by its opponents as little more than infanticide, and the proposed legislation would have prohibited it except when clearly needed to save the mother's life. Those who encouraged the president's veto of the bill insisted that this procedure is often the safest one for the woman. They believed that the proposed legislation violated the constitutionally guaranteed primacy of a woman's life and health during the third trimester of pregnancy. They further argued that late-term abortion is sometimes needed to avoid the birth of a child with serious congenital anomalies whose delivery threatens the mother's life, health, or reproductive capacities. Present at the White House ceremony were a number of women who testified to the need for this extreme medical option. One speaker made a poignant appeal to her own Jewish religious background as a factor in her decision to terminate her pregnancy when she learned that the child she was carrying had multiple serious heart and brain anomalies.

I mention this episode to indicate how divisive the debate over the "sanctity" versus the "quality" of life has become in our society. On the "sanctity-of-life" side of the debate are those who believe that human life at all its stages is of infinite value. [1] Life must be protected from the moment of conception through natural death, and any termination of life or hastening of death, whether before birth or at the end of life's span, is impermissible. Some "right to life" advocates who hold this view permit the termination of pregnancy where a mother's life is in danger on the grounds that it is reasonable to sacrifice one life to save another. Others, including many Roman Catholic ethicists, disagree, holding that one may never intentionally and directly take an innocent human life for whatever reason. As a rule, those who hold the "sanctity-of-life" position also reject proposals for euthanasia or physician-assisted suicide as well as the cessation of aggressive care or food and fluids in the cases of terminally ill, suffering, or permanently comatose patients.

On the other side of the debate are those who believe that "quality-of-life" considerations must enter into our thinking at each step of life's progression. The value of life resides not in its biological or physical status, but in the presence of abilities to think, feel, and relate to others. Those who hold this view maintain that qualitative evaluations justify graded distinctions in the moral status of life at various stages of development. They commonly apply this thinking to prenatal existence in order to justify pregnancy termination for various reasons. Some apply the same thinking to the neonatal period, arguing that the quality of life for some newborns is so poor as to justify cessation of aggressive care. Where adults are concerned, those who think this way see quality-of-life considerations playing a legitimate role in decisions to forego treatment or even expedite dying through self-administered or physician-administered lethal agents.

This distinction between quality of life and sanctity of life is one of the leading bioethical questions of our day. At its heart it involves major religious and philosophical questions, including how we weigh the protection and prolongation of biological human life against other human values. In view of this issue's importance, it is worth asking where Judaism stands. Does Jewish thinking favor a sanctity-of-life or quality-of-life approach?

In addressing this question, I must first make clear what I mean by Judaism. This term embraces a wide variety of people, communities, and a host of conceptual positions. In what follows, I focus on what the Orthodox tradition of Jewish religious law, *halakhah*, says on the matter of the sanctity versus the quality of life. The tradition of Jewish law is the centuries-old context for Jewish thinking about ethical problems, including many problems in biology and medicine. Although most modern Jews do not regard themselves as bound by halakhic norms, this tradition nevertheless remains a distinctively coherent *Jewish* contribution to our thinking about bioethical subjects. I am a Jew who does not heed every commandment of Torah. Nevertheless, I believe that classical Jewish normative thinking merits respect because the great rabbinic decisors, some of whom were physicians, often had profound insight into the demands of human moral existence. [2] Even when some of their specific enactments have been rendered obsolete by time, this moral wisdom remains apparent at the level of principle. As we face our own controversies about the sanctity or quality of life, therefore, it is worth examining the resources of this tradition for understanding modern issues.

Over the past two decades, a vigorous tradition of Orthodox Jewish bioethics has emerged. Scholars working in this area have produced attractively packaged, English-language compendia of Jewish bioethical teachings based on traditional talmudic and rabbinic sources. They also publish often in the pages of respected Orthodox journals like *Tradition*. One of the leading spokesman for contemporary Orthodox bioethics is Rabbi J. David Bleich, whose articles, books, and edited volumes gather together a host of opinions culled from contemporary Orthodox responsa and other similar sources. In what follows I shall focus mostly on Bleich's writings, although his positions are largely concordant with the majority of Orthodox bioethicists, including Rabbi Immanuel Jakobovits, whose 1975 book *Jewish Medical Ethics* inaugurated modern Orthodox thinking in this area. For many non-Orthodox Jews and for others interested in Jewish perspectives on biomedical ethics, the writings of Bleich and Jakobovits are often a natural first resort as they seek to understand Jewish thinking on medical ethics.

Anyone looking at the literature of Orthodox bioethics would quickly conclude that Judaism adheres to a staunch sanctity-of-life perspective. Bleich sums up this position when he says "Judaism teaches that human life is sacred from the moment of generation of genoplasm in the gonads until decomposition of the body after death." [3] This position is often traced to the biblical account of the creation of the world from a single person, Adam. Drawing on this, the talmudic tractate Sanhedrin declares that "whosoever preserves a single soul of Israel, Scripture ascribes [merit] to him as though he had preserved a complete world." [4] As Bleich and others point out, the value of a single life is given expression in traditional Jewish law by limits on individual autonomy in the control of one's life, by mandates for self-preservation, and by the teaching of *pikku'ah nefesh*, according to which virtually all ritual obligations must be set aside if needed to save a life.

Although Bleich's characterization of the Orthodox position is not unchallenged in Orthodox circles, it remains fairly representative of the view of Orthodox bioethicists on matters regarding the treatment of human life at its various stages. Despite this substantial consensus that Judaism espouses a sanctity-of-life position, however, I shall present a more nuanced and complex view. I hope to indicate that classical Jewish thinkers were deeply sensitive to qualitative considerations and a host of values competing with mere biological survival. Foremost among their other concerns was the minimization of suffering rather than the continuance of life itself. Applying this thinking to prenatal existence, they came up with a remarkably permissive set of norms governing reproductive behavior, especially abortion. They were also sometimes willing to apply this logic to decisions at the end of life, where cessation of treatment or active efforts to end life were options. To be sure, many of their rulings were made in a context of different technological and medical realities, which sometimes obscures the broad permissiveness of the tradition on these matters. Further complicating things is the fact that in some cases there is a range of classical views. Modern Orthodox bioethicists do not err in presenting one side of the picture, but there is often another side that deserves a hearing. What follows then is something of an oddity: an argument by a modern, secularized moral philosopher of Jewish background who is not a talmudic scholar to the effect that many skilled and devoted contemporary halakhists may not be right when they contend that classical Judaism espouses a strict "sanctity-of-life" position. Many aspects of this tradition, I maintain, fit better within a "quality-of-life" approach.

PRENATAL DECISION MAKING

With very few exceptions, most contemporary Orthodox bioethicists affirm that Judaism rigorously upholds the sanctity of prenatal human life and opposes abortion except when needed to preserve the mother's life. Their views differ little from those of conservative Roman Catholic or Protestant thinkers. Indeed, in national and international debates on abortion or such matters as fetal tissue or human embryo research, contemporary Orthodox bioethicists have occasionally made common cause with Catholic and Protestant opponents of these practices. During a recent international conference on bioethics sponsored by the Council of Europe, for example, a Jewish spokesman on a panel dealing with religious views of the human embryo urged a position broadly similar to that espoused by the representative of the Holy See. [5]

Orthodox bioethicists usually base their position on one talmudic passage, *Oholot* (7:6). [6] The text itself is very graphic and brings to mind our own recent debates about "partial-birth" abortions. It reads:

> If a woman is in hard travail, we cut up the child in her womb and bring it forth member by member, because her life comes before that of the child. But if the greater part has proceeded forth, one may not touch it, for one may not set aside one person's life for that of another.

At first sight, this text does not appear to support a strict sanctity-of-life position, such as that espoused by the Roman Catholic Church. To some extent, it admits a qualitative distinction between stages of human life. The preborn child, *Oholot* suggests, is not yet on a moral plane with its mother. Although Jewish thought normally hesitates to recommend the taking of one life to preserve another, on the principle that no one can claim that his blood is redder than another's, in this case the lesser status of the fetus dictates a preference for the mother. Jewish thinking here contrasts with the Roman Catholic position, where the full moral equivalence of the fetus and the mother and a ban on direct killing of a human being yield the conclusion that we must allow both mother and child to die. Judaism's strict priority on maternal over fetal life also leads to the conclusion that the choice to save the mother in such cases is mandatory. Because of the obligation to preserve a life, neither the mother nor the family may opt to risk her life to see the child born. In this respect, classical Jewish teaching, even in its most conservative interpretations, differs from Catholic and some Protestant thinking. [7]

This said, most contemporary Orthodox bioethicists stop here in their view of the permissibility of abortion. Most acknowledge only the smallest fraction of difference between prenatal and postnatal human life. They concede that the fetus may not have the moral status of born children or adults, but they believe that it nevertheless has substantial sanctity as a potential life, with the consequence that a pregnancy may be terminated only for the gravest of reasons. Their view is partly based on the fact that while *Oholot* requires abortion when the mother's life is in peril, the text says nothing about other justifying grounds for the procedure. May non-life-threatening maternal health considerations or the mother's emotional distress enter into our thinking about the allowability of abortion? What about problems in the child, such as genetic or congenital defects? To what extent are familial convenience or personal economic or career concerns legitimating reasons? On all these matters, *Oholot* is silent.

Proceeding from this silence, a tradition of halakhic scholarship to which most contemporary Orthodox bioethical writers belong interprets *Oholot* narrowly to imply that abortion is permitted only in cases where the mother's life is in peril—but not for lesser reasons. This reading of *Oholot* is also sometimes supported by an interpretation of Maimonides' commentary on the passage. Discussing this ruling, Maimonides explained that in such cases, the fetus may be likened to a pursuer (*rodef*) who places another's life in peril and who, according to Jewish law, may be killed without the defender's incurring the penalty of capital punishment. [8] Drawing on this discussion, some later commentators maintain that since the fetus is like an adult pursuer, its life may be taken only when another's life is endangered, but not for lesser reasons. On this account, virtually no quality-of-life considerations underlie the *Oholot* ruling. Mother and child are moral equals. Only the objective "aggression" of the child justifies taking its life in these circumstances.

This restrictive reading of *Oholot* figures substantially in the views of virtually all contemporary Orthodox Jewish bioethicists. The fact that these writers profoundly identify with this restrictive view on abortion can be illustrated with reference to the matter of prenatal diagnosis and abortion for genetic reasons. Clearly some of the most difficult decisions in medical ethics lie in this area. What are Jewish parents to do when they learn that the second trimester child the woman is carrying is affected by Tay-Sachs disease, a condition that will lead to inevitable neurological decline and death before five years of age? What are they to do in the face of other serious genetic disorders that cause acute suffering and disability?

To these and other questions, the writings of most of the leading Orthodox bioethicists today offer fairly straightforward answers. They insist that genetic considerations, in and of themselves, do not constitute a reason for deferring procreation or for permitting abortion. Since Jewish law teaches that life, whatever its quality or stage of development, is sacred, a pregnancy may be terminated only to save the mother's life. Abortion in these cases is halakhicly permitted only if the birth of a genetically deformed child would likely drive the mother to suicide. Where her mental stability is not at risk, the parents must welcome the child, no matter how serious its disorder. [9] It follows from this reasoning that abortion for any lesser reason is not permissible.

These views illustrate the extent to which these writers regard Judaism's adherence to the sanctity of prenatal life and the irrelevance of qualitative thinking in biomedical decision making. Not even a disease as horrible as Tay-Sachs persuades them to moderate their position. In view of this unbending rigor, it would be reasonable for the reader unfamiliar with Jewish law to conclude that the classical norms regarding abortion must be unambiguous and immutable. But this is not at all the case. If anything, the bulk of the early halakhic tradition supports a view that makes sharp distinctions between human life in its developing stages.

The foundation of halakhic reasoning in this area is Exodus 21:22, where killing of the fetus by a third party is regarded as a tort (primarily against the father) and not as an act of homicide. This text is explained by later writers, including the important commentator Rashi, in terms of the fact that the fetus is not a *nefesh*, a living person in the juridical or moral sense. [10] Commentators expanded on this by categorizing the child before birth as technically "a part of the mother's body." [11] Before its birth it is *lav nefesh hu*, not a person. [12] This halakhic estimate of fetal life, incidentally, has nothing to do with rabbinic ideas of ensoulment, which comprise a spectrum of quite different views. [13] Neither speculative material on the origin of personhood, nor haggadic, imaginative narrative discussions of uterine life are normative, but the authoritative biblical text.

This classical talmudic attitude toward prenatal life is also dramatically evidenced by a text which is usually neglected or touched on only in passing by contemporary Orthodox Jewish bioethicists. This text, in tractate 'Arakin (7a), establishes norms for the execution of a woman who has been convicted of a capital crime but who is found to be pregnant after her trial was concluded. The question before the sages is whether the execution might be delayed— even for a matter of hours—to allow the child to be born. 'Arakin's answer is blunt:

> If a woman is about to be executed, one does not wait for her until she gives birth: But if she had already sat on the birthstool, one waits for her until she gives birth.

In the Gemara or commentary that follows this authoritative text of oral law (Mishnah), a reason for the ruling is given:

> But that is self-evident, for it is her body!—It is necessary to teach it for one might have assumed since Scripture says: "According as the woman's husband shall lay upon him"(Exodus 21:22), that it [the unborn child] is the husband's property, of which he should not be deprived, therefore we are informed [that it is not so].

What this text makes clear is that for classical rabbinic thinking, informed by its biblical foundations, the moral value of the fetus and its worth to the father are both dramatically subordinated to the suffering of the woman. A contrast here with both Roman and Islamic law is useful. In Roman law, a woman's execution is delayed because she is the bearer of valuable materiel: a future citizen of the Roman state. Her feelings do not count. In Islamic law, the life of the fetus is given priority over any additional suffering the woman may undergo in the possibly long wait for her execution. Not so in Jewish law. 'Arakin tells us that her well-being, even in this desperate circumstance, is not subordinated to her role as a reproductive entity or to any claims of the fetus's life.

Lest we doubt this, the text concludes with the ruling that, in such cases, it is appropriate to strike the condemned woman on the abdomen shortly before the execution in order to kill the child. This is done, the rabbis tell us, to prevent her disgrace (*nivvul*) should a living child emerge from her body during the execution. Fetal life, even at the moments near birth, has less of a claim on us than the preservation of a woman's dignity. The governing principle here is that her pain should be the first consideration (*tza'ara d'gufah kadim*). [14]

This is a gruesome text. Small wonder it is ignored even by modern Jewish proponents of the right of abortion. However, we must keep in mind the real intent of the teaching here: in a context where capital punishment is taken for granted, the sages are clearly demonstrating their concern for the mother rather than for the fetus. Saving the fetus's life does not justify inflicting even a few more hours of suffering on her. Likewise, the prospect of her disgrace bulks larger in the sages' view than any claims of prenatal life. [15]

This text was never abandoned by the halakhic tradition. Among other things, it plays a part in a ruling by the eighteenth century rabbi Jacob Emden, which permitted an adulteress to conceal her crime by having an abortion. Emden reasoned that if the woman's crime became known, she would be convicted of a capital offense and the child would be dead in any case. Hence the woman might seek to save her life by having an abortion. [16] Beyond this, Emden and others drew upon the concepts underlying the classical ruling to conclude that a woman might have an abortion in any case of 'great pain'. More recently, Emden's thinking was used by the great Israeli decisor Rabbi Eliezer Waldenberg in a ruling that permitted selective abortion where the fetus is likely to be genetically diseased. [17] Following Emden, a small number of commentators have also legitimated abortion in instances of even 'slight need' on the mother's part. These and other texts evidence what Mark Washofsky calls "the fluidity of Jewish legal discussion on abortion." [18]

Beyond this issue, the classical halakhic tradition actually introduces a complex graded perception of the moral status of early human life in its various stages of development. For example, the rabbis regarded the embryo during the first forty days of pregnancy as almost without moral status or value, judging it, in their words, to be "mere fluid." [19] As a pregnancy developed, the fetus presumably gained greater moral weight, but rabbinic qualitative reasoning did not abate. The standard teaching was that a stillborn child at any stage does not require burial, a significant denial of status in this highly ritualized tradition. Full mourning rituals are also withheld from a newborn who dies before thirty days of age. This partly reflects halakhic uncertainty over whether the newborn represents a completed pregnancy. It may also evidence the belief that, while any loss of a child is traumatic for parents, the death of one with whom a relationship has not yet been fully established is of lesser moral importance.

This graded appreciation of the developing moral status of human life, especially during its prenatal stages, is deeply relevant to some of the most important bioethics debates of our day. Several years ago, I served on the National Institutes of Health's Human Embryo Research Panel. The charge to this diverse group of scientists, ethicists, and policymakers was to furnish guidelines for future federally funded research on the preimplantation human embryo, the embryo as it is encountered during procedures of *in vitro* fertilization. From the beginning of our work, the panel had to answer the question of whether it is morally permissible to accord a lesser moral status to the human embryo during the first two weeks of development, the period that is most important for current research. We concluded that aspects of the early preimplantation embryo, its lack of cell differentiation, absence of completed individuation (early embryos can twin, and twins can recombine into single-tons), and the very high natural rate of embryo loss in early pregnancy, warrant a moral distinction between the preimplantation embryo and the later fetus. On this basis, and because we privileged the needs of children and adults who might benefit from research, we permitted some kinds of carefully regulated embryo research. [20] Our conclusions were strenuously resisted by a coalition of Roman Catholic and conservative Protestant groups that had an influential role in shaping later congressional rejection of our proposals.

In this connection, I must observe that classical Jewish thinking broadly conforms to the reasoning of our panel. The judgment that the very early embryo is "mere fluid" is a sound appreciation of the relative formlessness, lack of humanly relevant qualities, and lack of parental emotional attachment that are morally significant at this stage of pregnancy, when most women do not even know they are pregnant. That the early rabbis could acknowledge this and could preserve a clear sense that human life is not equally sacred at all its stages is something that must not be lost in our current debates. We must not conclude that all biblically based religions are committed to the kind of vitalism that has become the hallmark of many traditions today. To the extent that halakhic reasoning holds out a markedly different view of the moral status of the early embryo than is present, say, in current Catholic or evangelical Protestant thought, the question also arises for public policy of whether American law should privilege some religiously derived views over another.

DECISION MAKING AT THE END OF LIFE

When we turn to end-of-life decision making and the question of sanctity versus quality of life, the gap between the positions espoused by contemporary Orthodox bioethicists and the classical rabbinic tradition is less extreme.

Contemporary Orthodox commentators are right to report that classical sources are wary about any qualitative judgments that might lead to a hastening of human death. Judaism has always placed great value on respect and compassion for human beings, whatever their status or condition. This compassion extends to those who are desperately ill or whose expectation of life is short. In classical sources, this sometimes justifies heroic lifesaving measures and always counsels against behavior that conveys to the dying anything less than a message of full compassion. Nevertheless, I believe that some modern Orthodox writers fail to pick up important aspects of classical teachings, aspects that have become more important in our changed technological and medical environment.

As a rule, these writers hold to the view that Judaism is deeply opposed to the direct killing of suffering or dying patients, what is usually called "active euthanasia," as well as almost all forms of cessation of aggressive therapy or lifesaving efforts, sometimes called "passive euthanasia," no matter how ill or how much in pain the patient may be. They find support for these conclusions in a number of talmudic texts. The classical rabbis ruled, for example, that efforts on the Sabbath to free a person buried under the rubble of a collapsed building must be continued even if the victim is so injured that he cannot live more than a short time. [21] It was also held that anyone who killed a child while it was falling from a high roof would, in principle, be regarded as a murderer, even if the child would otherwise have died immediately. [22]

Drawing on these teachings, Rabbi Bleich asserts categorically that "the quality of life that is preserved is . . . never a factor to be taken into consideration" in Jewish teaching. [23] Bleich argues that Judaism rejects the Roman Catholic distinction between ordinary and extraordinary, or proportionate and disproportionate, means. He contends that any medication or procedure needed to sustain life must be employed, and he categorically rejects as permissible for the devout Jew any sort of "living will" in which the patient stipulates a limit to medical care *in extremis*. [24] The obligation to sustain life obtains even if the injured person has only moments remaining. A similar view is expressed by Rabbi Immanuel Jakobovits. [25] As for the prolonged or intensified suffering experienced by the dying patient as a result of aggressive medical efforts, these writers tend to view this in providential terms, as part of our divinely appointed life course which we may not seek to evade. Severe terminal disease must be accepted as "a manifestation of providence designed to induce introspection and repentance." [26] However, this does not rule out the use of analgesics like opium or heroin to relieve pain for a dying patient, even if these medications might have the side-effect of hastening death. [27]

Apart from this use of palliative agents, the only exception to aggressive therapy these writers find in the classical tradition arises in the case of the *goses*, a patient who has already entered the dying process. Classical texts define the *goses* as one on the very brink of death: his breathing is labored, his chest "narrows" and he brings up "a secretion" in his throat. [28] While such patients are to be treated with extreme care—they must not be jostled, placed on the ground, or otherwise disturbed [29]—and while no active efforts may be made to hasten their death, it was regarded as permissible to remove certain 'impediments' to their dying. Thus, one classical source held that anything which rivets the soul's attentions—such as a bit of salt on the tongue or the noise of a wood chopper in the vicinity—might be removed or stopped in order allow the patient to die. [30] In an effort to lend more precision to this concept, Rabbi Bleich draws on what he believes to be the relevant classical sources to conclude that such a patient is one who cannot survive for more than seventy-two hours. [31] Any patient, no matter what his condition, who can survive longer than this is not a *goses* and hence must receive unceasing medical care. In a recent discussion, Bleich further argues that *gessisah*, the state of being a *goses*, is not determined by a patient's ability to survive for seventy-two hours solely by natural means unaided by medical interventions. Rather, for one to be declared a *goses*, it must be shown that "the state is not only irreversible but also not prolongable even by artificial means." Thus, according to Bleich, a comatose patient whose biological functioning can be maintained indefinitely by a ventilator, total parenteral nutrition, dialysis, surgically implanted shunts, or antibiotics is not a *goses*.

I am confident that even the most conservative classical rabbis who defined the status of the *goses* would be shocked by this mode of reasoning. Certainly, their concepts of compassion for the dying and respect for basic human dignity did not extend to the virtually unending preservation of biological functioning that technology now makes possible. In an era when the causes of death were not well understood and recovery from even serious diseases was possible, the rabbis urged perseverance in reasonable efforts to save a life. Nevertheless, when it was clear that only death and suffering were in prospect, they counseled gentleness and an end to active interventions. This is the meaning of the state of *gessisah*. To fixate on the inability to prolong life for at least seventy-two hours (by any means) as the sole criterion for discontinuing aggressive interventions, is to take these rulings out of their original biomedical context and to omit entirely the other value considerations that led the rabbis to them.

There is also the question of how we are to interpret some of the other key textual supports on which the modern Orthodox interpreters rely. Take for example the appeal to the talmudic teaching that efforts on the Sabbath to free a person buried under the rubble of a building must be continued even if the victim is so injured that he cannot live more than a short time.

This is a reasonable ruling. In the wake of the tragic episodes at the federal building in Oklahoma City or U.S. embassy bombings in Africa, we can appreciate the deep respect for human life that is involved in unsparing efforts to save someone trapped in this way. Anything less than this, the mere prospect of leaving someone to the despair of abandonment in such circumstances, is ethically unthinkable. When we add the consideration that in these situations there is the chance, however small, that a fully functional person may be rescued, talmudic teaching makes perfect sense. If we extrapolate this, as the classical rabbis sometimes did, to medical efforts, this position also makes sense. Compared with us, our forebears had a relatively poor understanding of the course of disease. Spontaneous recoveries from seemingly fatal conditions were not uncommon, and, in any case, desperate but compassionate efforts to sustain life were usually self-limiting and checked by nature's irrevocable course.

How different this is from any of our end-of-life medical decisions today where we both know the fatal outcome with certainty and can forestall it indefinitely. Some years ago, a ninety-four-year-old relative of mine fell while strolling in the forest and struck his head. Found unconscious, he was hospitalized, but he never recovered consciousness and progressively lost function in vital organs. After two weeks of dialysis with no return of kidney function despite repeated efforts to wean him from the machines, the decision arrived as to whether we should continue aggressive efforts to keep him alive. The family chose not to do so, and the old man died peacefully a short while later. My relative was not a *goses* in Rabbi Bleich's terms. He was not immanently and unavoidably dying. But a humane decision was made to cease rescue efforts and to allow him to die peacefully. Surely it is inappropriate to liken him to a sick but potentially viable patient in the sixth or thirteenth century. Surely it is mistaken to compare his situation with the condition of someone trapped in the rubble of a building. Unfortunately, too much contemporary Orthodox bioethics evidences failures of moral imagination of this sort. Too often, classical halakhic texts displaying keen moral insight and compassion *in the context of their day* are rigidly applied to dramatically altered circumstances. The result is a sanctity-of-life position that is out of touch with other, equally important, currents of classical Jewish thought.

The problem goes deeper than this. Sometimes, contemporary Orthodox bioethicists ignore or misinterpret talmudic texts that applaud efforts to hasten the demise of desperately ill, suffering, or terminal patients. For example, several texts approve of praying for divine intervention to end a course of desperate suffering. One text describes an incident where a host of rabbis were praying for the life of Judah the Prince, who lay dying with a painful gastrointestinal disorder. [32] Amidst the uproar, a simple serving girl, taking note of the dying sage's suffering, asks God to bring it to an end. The text goes on to report that she then accidentally dropped a pitcher on the ground, startling the rabbis and momentarily causing them to stop praying. With this, the soul of the dying man departed. Noteworthy here are the clear approval of the serving girl's actions and the implicit criticism directed at the rabbis' unthinking efforts to sustain life beyond reasonable limits.

It may be argued that mention of prayer in these cases has little relevance to the cessation of active medical care, since in the case of prayer, it is God, not human beings, who acts to bring life to an end. But this misses the fact that for the rabbis, prayer was just as efficacious as medical measures, which were themselves viewed as working only with divine cooperation. [33] By permitting the cessation of prayer and allowing prayers for a patient's demise, the texts were telling us that it is sometimes reasonable to intentionally try to bring life of very poor quality more rapidly to an end. [34] The suffering from which relief might be requested by prayer also included that arising from purely psychological considerations. Several talmudic texts record with approbation instances of elderly individuals who pray for death as an escape from the fatigue, loneliness, or the depression of old age. [35]

Particularly interesting in terms of end-of-life decision making is a famous talmudic passage recounting the martyrdom of Rabbi Hanina ben T[e]radyon. [36] The Romans had placed the sage in a fire, and to prolong his agony they had covered his chest with damp tufts of wool. According to the talmudic account, the rabbi's disciples pleaded with him to open his mouth wide so that he might quickly be asphyxiated by the smoke. Refusing this request on the grounds that it would constitute suicide, the rabbi replied, "Only He Who gave life can take it away; I may not do it myself."

At this point, we read that one of the Roman executioners, taking pity on the rabbi, "raised the flame and removed the tufts of wool from over his heart," permitting the rabbi's soul to depart. The narrative goes on to tell us that because of this act of mercy, the executioner "went straight to heaven when he died." Rabbi Judah the Prince spoke enviously of him, observing that while some of us strive throughout our lifetimes to earn a place in the world to come, others, like this good Roman, earn a place there in a single moment of righteousness.

Although this text portrays the saintly sage as upholding the Judaic aversion to suicide, and may even be read as commending a pious, but not necessarily mandatory, willingness to acquiesce to suffering at life's end, it also boldly upholds efforts to hasten death in at least two different ways: first, by removing impediments that slow a painful and certain dying process (the damp tufts of wool); and, second, by actively taking measures to accelerate dying (raising the flames). Even if one tries to argue that the executioner's intensifying of the fire merely put an end to the unnatural and tortured death that the Romans were inflicting on the rabbi, it remains true that his intervention killed the rabbi more quickly. This supports the claim that the classical sages accepted as morally praiseworthy at least some lethal interventions aimed at putting an end to a dying person's suffering. [37] Despite the views of many modern Orthodox interpreters, therefore, there exists a significant element in Jewish teaching not opposed to active killing and that supports the view that the relief of suffering can sometimes take priority over the protection or continuance of biological human existence.

Not all modern halakhicly based thinking in bioethics is as unimaginative on these matters as I have suggested. Some of the most penetrating rabbinic thinkers have recognized that new technical and scientific realities compel a change in the application of at least some traditional rules. For example, in the mid-1980s, Rabbi Moshe Feinstein, perhaps the leading rabbinic decisor of his generation, admitted modern definitions of brain death to Orthodox Jewish thinking. He did so, among other things, by making ingenuous appeal to traditional rulings that stipulated death in slaughtered animals as involving decapitation. [38] Feinstein's thinking helped counter a then prevalent tradition of Orthodox scholarship that would entirely ignore technological advances and insist on maintaining the traditional criteria of cessation of respiratory and cardiac function, however sustained, as a requirement for a declaration of death. Recently, some Orthodox bioethicists influenced by Feinstein, including Dr. Fred Rosner and Rabbi Moshe Tendler, have emphasized his permissions for cessation of aggressive treatment of terminally ill patients. Rosner and Tendler have also acknowledged those aspects of Jewish thinking about end-of-life decision making that together make up a "quality-of-life" perspective. [39]

Thus Orthodox bioethics is not monolithically committed to a vitalistic, sanctity-of-life view, and change is occurring as an appreciation of new medical realities penetrates traditional circles. Nevertheless, in some quarters change is very slow, and elsewhere one can even detect a deliberate retreat from more permissive classical Jewish positions as Jewish thinkers strive to show themselves as no less forceful than conservative Christians in demonstrating their opposition to the moral laxity of modernity. [40] In the area of reproductive decision making, these instincts are also impelled by the pronatalist commitments of some Orthodox Jewish groups. [41]

Nevertheless, these traditionalist thinkers do not represent the tradition in its full light. Jews and non-Jews, seeking to understand the tradition of Jewish thinking about biomedical ethics, should be warned to delve more deeply into the classical sources and be wary about some modern Orthodox presentations of the tradition. Although classical Judaism deeply valued human life and partly created a great tradition of Jewish medicine for this very reason, Jewish thinkers always recognized that it is not biological existence that counts, but the values that life is meant to sustain and support. When these values are threatened or degraded by biological existence, the classical texts do not hesitate to suggest that it is not life, but the nature and quality of that life that come first.

As I imagine the great rabbis who formed the talmudic tradition facing biomedical ethical choices in our day, I feel confident that they would come to certain conclusions. With reference to the beginning of life, I have little doubt that they would strive to preserve the life and health of pregnant women over any claims, however sentimentally presented, that might be made on behalf of the embryo or fetus. To the extent that embryo extraction for late-term abortion, the procedure opponents call partial-birth abortion, is even marginally superior as a technique for preserving the life and health of the mother, I believe the rabbis would conclude that this procedure is required by Jewish law. They would base this opinion on the teaching that the mother's pain comes first and that human life is not equally sacred at all stages of development: that, until its birth, the fetus *lav nefesh hu*, is not a person.

As far as end-of-life decision making is concerned, the sages would surely urge compassionate care for the sick and employment of even heroic efforts to restore functional life. However, on the grounds that death is sometimes preferable to life marked by extreme physical or psychological suffering, I believe they would urge forbearance from pointless medical interventions and the mere prolongation of biological existence in terminal patients or those experiencing intractable pain. I am less sure how they would view active euthanasia or physician-assisted suicide. Because of the very positive valuation they placed on life and their aversion to killing, the rabbis would probably be uncomfortable with these practices. Recent Jewish experience with the Nazi employment of active euthanasia as a prelude to genocide would also lead them to counsel great caution. [42] Nevertheless, it is not clear to me that they would unalterably oppose even active efforts to end life in extreme cases of suffering. A tradition that promised heavenly reward to a compassionate Roman executioner might find a place in the world to come for Dr. Kevorkian.

NOTES

1. For a discussion of various definitions and understandings of quality and sanctity of life, see James J. Walters, "Quality of Life in Clinical Decisions," in *Encyclopedia of Bioethics*, vol. 3 (New York: Macmillan, 1995): 1352–58.

2. Louis E. Newman would replace this text-based, precedent-seeking approach to talmudic texts, with a more open-textured admission that all legal resources are interpreted in terms of contemporary needs and experience. See his "Woodchoppers and Respirators: The Problem of Interpretation in Contemporary Jewish Ethics," in Elliot N. Dorff and Louis E. Newman, eds., *Contemporary Jewish Ethics and Morality* (New York: Oxford University Press, 1995): 140–60. Against Newman, I believe that authoritative texts point to abiding ways of approaching bioethical issues. The effort should be made to understand them, however, in terms of the contexts in which they were developed and applied.

3. J. David Bleich, "Survey of Recent Halakhic Periodical Literature: Treatment of the Terminally Ill," *Tradition*, vol. 24, no. 4 (1989): 71.

4. Tractate Sanhedrin, *Babylonian Talmud*, 37a.

5. B. Kannovitch, "Une Réflection Juive sur 'La Nature et le Status de L'Embryon Humain'." Paper presented at the 3rd Symposium on Bioethics: Medically-Assisted Procreation and the Protection of the Human Embryo. Council of Europe. Strasbourg, December 15–18, 1996.

6. Tractate Sanhedrin, *Babylonian Talmud*, 74a.

7. Although not constrained by the Catholic prohibition on direct killing, conservative Protestant thinkers might permit a mother to risk or sacrifice her life to save her preborn child. Jewish law, with its requirement to preserve one's life and its lesser valuation of the fetus, removes this option.

8. The Code of Maimonides in the *Mishneh Torah*, 19 vols. (New Haven: Yale University Press, 1949): vol. 11: 196.

9. J. David Bleich, *Judaism and Healing* (New York: Ktav, 1981): 103–08; Fred Rosner and J. David Bleich, eds., *Jewish Bioethics* (New York: Sanhedrin Press, 1979): 123f., 160f.

10. Rashi, *Pentateuch with Commentary*, Horeb edition (Berlin, 1928), Sanhedrin, 7b.

11. Tractate Hulin, *Babylonian Talmud*, 58 and tractate Gittin, 23b.

12. David Feldman, "Abortion, Religious Traditions, Jewish Perspectives," in *Encyclopedia of Bioethics*, vol. 1: 26–29.

13. Feldman, "Abortion, Religious Traditions, Jewish Perspectives," 27f. Also Feldman, *Marital Relations, Birth Control and Abortion in Jewish Law* (New York: Schocken Books, 1974): 271–75.

14. Feldman, "Abortion, Religious Traditions, Jewish Perspectives," 28.

15. The woman-centered nature of some classical Jewish bioethics is signaled by Dena S. Davis, "Beyond Rabbi Hiyya's Wife: Women's Voices in Jewish Bioethics," *Second Opinion* 16 (1991): 10–31.

16. Feldman, "Abortion, Religious Traditions, Jewish Perspectives," 28; Feldman, *Marital Relations*, 288f.; also, David Sinclair, "The Legal Basis for the Prohibition on Abortion in Jewish Law," in the *Israel Law Review* 15 (1980): 109–30.

17. David Sinclair, "The Legal Basis for the Prohibition on Abortion in Jewish Law," 124f.

18. "Abortion and the Halakhic Conversation: A Liberal Perspective" in *The Fetus and Fertility in Jewish Law: Essays and Responsa*, Walter Jacobs and Moshe Zemer, eds. (Pittsburgh and Tel Aviv: Frehof Institute of Progressive Halakhah, 1995): 47. Mark Washofsky emphasizes the role of an earlier decisor than Emden, Rabbi Yosef Trani, in the tradition of lenient rulings stemming from the Arakin text and Rashi.

19. Tractate Yebamoth, *Babylonian Talmud,* 69b, tractate Niddin, *Babylonian Talmud,* 3, 7, 30b.

20. *National Institutes of Health: Report of the Human Embryo Research Panel* (Bethesda, Md.: National Institutes of Health, September 27, 1994).

21. Joseph Karo, *Shulhan 'Arukh,* Romm, ed., (Vilna, 1911); *Orah Hayyim* 329: 4.

22. Tractate Baba Kamma, *Babylonian Talmud,* 26b.

23. Bleich, "Survey of Recent Halakhic Periodical Literature," 57.

24. Bleich, "Survey of Recent Halakhic Peiodical Literature," 61. See also his *Judaism and Healing,* 139.

25. Immanuel Jakobovits, *Jewish Medical Ethics* (New York: Bloch, 1975): 276.

26. Bleich, "Survey of Recent Halakhic Periodical Literature," 60.

27. Bleich, "Survey of Recent Halakhic Periodical Literature," 62. Jakobovits, *Jewish Medical Ethics,* 276.

28. Bleich, "Survey of Recent Halakhic Periodical Literature," 63.

29. Moses Maimonides, *The Code of Maimonides* 14: 174.

30. Jakobovits, *Jewish Medical Ethics,* 123.

31. Bleich, *Judaism and Healing,* 141.

32. Tractate Ketubot, *Babylonian Talmud,* 104a.

33. Jakobovits, *Jewish Medical Ethics,* 16.

34. The view that rabbinic permissions of prayer for the patient's death provide a talmudic precedent for active euthanasia is defended by Byron Sherwin, "A View of Euthanasia," Dorff and Newman, eds., *Contemporary Jewish Ethics and Morality,* 363–81.

35. See, for example, the story of the Sage Honi (tractate Taanit, *Babylonian Talmud,* 23a); of the old men of the city of Luz (tractate Sotah, *Babylonian Talmud,* 46b); and the Midrashic tale of the very old woman wishing to die who came to Rabbi Yose ben Halafta and was instructed to cease her life-sustaining practice of twice-a-day prayer in the synagogue (*Proverbs Rabbah* 8). This episode is quoted by Byron Sherwin, "A View of Euthanasia," 371.

36. Tractate Avodah Zarah, *Babylonian Talmud,* 18a.

37. This point is made by Baruch Brody, "A Historical Introduction to Jewish Casuistry on Suicide and Euthanasia," *Suicide and Euthanasia: Historical and Contemporary Themes,* Baruch Brody, ed. (Dordrecht: Kluwer Academic Publishers, 1989): 39–75.

38. For one account of Rabbi Feinstein's innovative decisions, see Fred Rosner, "Rabbi Moshe Feinstein on the Treatment of the Terminally Ill," in *Judaism* 37 (Spring 1988): 188–89. Feinstein's use of reasoning by analogy in the case of definitions of death does not, however, have a parallel in his rulings on abortion which follow the modern, very restrictive tradition of other Orthodox halakhists. For a discussion of Feinstein's reasoning in this area, see Washofsky, "Abortion and Halakhic Conversation," 51–56.

39. Fred Rosner, "Quality and Sanctity of Life in the Talmud and Mishnah," in *Tradition,* vol. 28, no. 1 (1993): 18–27.

40. David Sinclair argues that the effort to match conservative Christian positions in moral strictness plays a role in Orthodox Jewish positions on sexuality and abortion. See his "The Legal Basis for the Prohibition on Abortion in Jewish Law," 126f. Washofsky, "Abortion and the Halakhic Conversation," emphasizes how much the fear of authorizing licentious sexual behavior has motivated the very stringent rulings on abortion by modern Orthodox halakhists.

41. David Feldman, "Population Ethics, Religious Traditions, Jewish Perspectives," *Encyclopedia of Bioethics*, vol. 4: 1981–85; Sandra B. Lubarsky, "Judaism and the Justification of Abortion for Nonmedical Reasons," in Dorff and Newman, eds., *Contemporary Jewish Ethics and Morality*: 396.

42. Arthur I. Eidelman, "Care of Critically Ill Newborns: The Israeli Experience," *The Journal of Legal Medicine* 16 (1995): 256.

The Jewish Approach to Living and Dying

Shimon Glick, M.D.

When presenting "Jewish attitudes" to any subject, it is appropriate to specify in advance what specific position is represented within the spectrum of extant Jewish positions. Israeli governments have fallen over the definition of "who is a Jew." Various Israeli supreme court justices have, in their published decisions, defined Judaism's core values in diametrically opposing ways. Jews everywhere today live in pluralistic societies, and many different voices claim to speak for Judaism.

The "Jewish attitude" in the present paper does not refer to the results of a poll among bagel-eating individuals with a name identifiable as being of middle-European Jewish origin. Rather, it refers to those individuals who consciously govern their lives by the tenets of their faith and who actively seek out Jewish values to guide their actions. These individuals, while clearly a minority among ethnic Jews, to my mind compose the group whose voice can be appropriately said to represent the "Jewish attitude."

The majority of these Jews are what are commonly referred to as Orthodox, and therefore I feel no need to apologize, or be defensive, about using these values as representative of Judaism. Furthermore, even those who do not identify as Orthodox, if they are serious about using Judaism's values to guide their decisions, must ultimately fall back on the classic Jewish sources, no matter how differently they are interpreted—and there is certainly room for various interpretations. These sources represent probably the longest unbroken tradition in bioethics which is still followed by its adherents. Former Israeli supreme court justice and talmudic scholar Menahem Elon estimates that there are over three hundred thousand halakhic responsa, a veritable treasure of casuistic literature on which all Jewish scholars of whatever persuasion are dependent. Before referring to actual Jewish texts, I want to comment about Jewish culture, with regard to attitudes towards life and death.

The task of defining Jewish culture is no less difficult. Russian Jewish culture differs from Moroccan Jewish culture, which in turn differs from

American or Yemenite Jewish culture. But each of these, in turn, differs from the specific non-Jewish culture that surrounds it. In Israel we have a blend of multiple Jewish cultures—mixed, but not homogenized, into a unique Israeli blend of Jewish culture, which includes, perhaps very importantly for bioethics, the post-Holocaust impact. There is, I believe, a commonality—a Jewish ethos that can be extracted from these diverse Jewish cultural expressions.

I remember distinctly a visit of mine as a lecturer at the University of Manitoba School of Medicine in the 1960s when the chairman of the department of medicine there asked me whether I had an explanation for his observation among the physicians in his department. He had noted that the Jewish physicians tried much harder in treating their patients and gave up much later in the struggle for saving lives than did their Christian counterparts. At that time I had no answer for him, nor could I confirm the validity of his observation. But I now believe that this perceptive clinician and educator did identify correctly an essential element of the Jewish ethos—a strong emphasis on life. This life ethos is reflected also in a number of other manifestations, including perhaps the impressive overrepresentation of Jews in the medical profession in almost all societies and eras. Other expressions of this culture include the relatively high percentage of Israeli patients on dialysis as compared to wealthier countries, the Israeli policy of placing physicians virtually on the front line in the battlefield in order to enhance the chances of saving the lives of wounded soldiers, and the overrepresentation of Israeli patients in transplantation centers around the world. Finally, there are a myriad of jokes confirming the perhaps exaggerated emphasis on life in the Jewish value system.

The Jewish culture is strongly pro-life, probably more so than its daughter religions, Christianity and Islam. This culture, even among avowedly secular Jews, is rooted in several thousand years of Jewish tradition and is religious in origin.

It is best expressed by the Mishnah in Sanhedrin: [1]

> Therefore was Adam created as a single individual—to teach us that one who destroys a single life is as if he destroys an entire world. And he who saves a single life is as if he saved an entire world. And so that one man should not say to his fellow man, "My father is greater than yours."

This statement in the Mishnah is responsible for what I call the "mythology" of the infinite value of human life; that is, that every life is of equal and infinite value, that even a moment of life is equivalent to longer periods of life, and that no value whatever is placed on the quality of life. I do not use the word "mythology" in a pejorative sense, nor do I wish to denigrate this principle which does bear a powerful and important message. But clearly no recognized halakhic authority prescribes a course of action in full accord with that phrase. Otherwise we would not permit anyone to die without an attempt at resuscitation and without attachment to a respirator, even if only for a few minutes. But the message, nevertheless, is clear and unequivocal. Life is of enormous significance. We dare not deliberately extinguish even a brief moment of life, even if this life is of poor quality. This is a valid and valuable myth which characterizes Jewish tradition.

Nevertheless, there is a dialectic here. On the one hand, life has intrinsic value, independent of what can be accomplished, and we are cautioned not to trifle with even tiny quanta of life, even if to our mortal perception this life serves no obvious purpose. Life is a precious divine gift of great intrinsic value—but it is also of instrumental value. Man is placed on earth to serve his Creator. The Jewish religion is one in which deeds are emphasized more so than merely beliefs. In the words of the Talmud: "One hour of good deeds is worth more than all of the world to come." [2] One may exploit even the shortest life opportunity to utter another amen, to say a prayer, to give a coin to a poor man, or to say a kind word to a distressed neighbor. Thus even in the area of the duty to save another's life, on the one hand some sages give a pragmatic rationale for the mandate to violate the Sabbath. "Violate a single Sabbath so that he may be enabled to keep many subsequent Sabbaths." [3] But on the other hand, the duty to violate the Sabbath takes precedence even if the patient is comatose and does not stand a chance to live beyond the moment, and certainly he will not be able to keep subsequent Sabbaths.

In spite of this unequivocal premium placed on human life, it is important to emphasize that life itself is not an absolute, nor even the ultimate highest value in Jewish tradition. The Torah commands us at times to sacrifice our own lives for higher values: for example, when one is faced with the forced violation of one of three cardinal sins (idol worship, murder, forbidden sexual relations) or at times when sacrifice of one's life is a matter of *kiddush hashem* (sanctification of God's name). The Torah also mandates the taking of human life, capital punishment, although only under very stringent limitations. Wars too are permitted, again only under certain clearly specified conditions. The command "*lo tirzakh*" in the Ten Commandments is not generally translated in Jewish sources as "do not kill," as it is in the King James Bible translation, but rather as "do not murder." There are times when taking a life is not just permitted, but even required.

There are several other aspects of the Jewish tradition that bear on the subject which should be mentioned. The Jewish physician-patient relationship, unlike that in the United States and some other Western countries, is not what Baruch Brody calls the contract type [4]—i.e., a totally voluntary relationship under which the physician agrees to undertake the care of a patient and the patient may or may not seek medical attention. The physician has a duty to help any patient who needs his assistance. This obligation is derived variously from several biblical ordinances, such as "Do not stand idly by your friend's blood" [5] and "You shall return it to him" [6]—the latter referring to the obligation to return a person's lost object and extended to include lost health.

The characteristic American slogan, "mind your own business," expressing a laissez-faire, individualistic attitude towards one's neighbour is not part of the Jewish tradition. The Jewish attitude may justifiably be termed paternalism, if you will, but in its positive, rather than in its commonly used pejorative connotation. Just as I would care deeply if one of my own children was sick and was headed for a disastrous decision, so too am I concerned about my patient, and I am obligated to help him/her in distress. Autonomy, the virtually unlimited right of a person to dispose of one's body as he/she sees fit, with no restrictions, is foreign to our tradition. Man is but a custodian of his body—bound by the ground rules imposed upon him by the Creator and ultimate owner of the body—the Almighty. In the West the last few decades have witnessed the rise of autonomy to the top of the list of ethical values, to the point that it often takes precedence over almost all other values. In our tradition, while there is more recognition of autonomy than is commonly believed, it certainly is far more limited than in the secular West. There is relative unanimity in the recent Jewish tradition that it is mandatory for a person to seek medical attention for any major illness and that it is equally mandatory to follow expert medical advice—particularly if a potential danger to life exists.

Suicide is unequivocally condemned in the Jewish halakhic literature, and the strictures prescribed in the *halakhah* about the burial, the treatment of the bodies, and the rules of mourning for those who have committed suicide are quite harsh and even seemingly cruel—particularly when one takes into account that those who suffer from this stance are the surviving family, who obviously have already suffered severely.

Yet side by side with the unequivocal condemnation of those who commit suicide, one can find another thread throughout history, from the Tanach to our own day. There are repeated attempts to find extenuating circumstances to mitigate the harsh attitudes towards suicide. In contrast with the strict uncompromising theory, the practice, as guided by the rabbis in dealing with individual cases in their communities, was usually much more understanding and forgiving. Rabbis went out of their way to unearth the most tenuous extenuating circumstances to permit the suicide's body to be treated respectfully and not ostracized. This is a fascinating and illuminating insight into the nuanced application of rabbinic law to meet the needs of the individual and of the circumstances. Interestingly enough, with the dramatic increase in societal approval of suicide and the rise in the rate of suicide in the West, Rabbi Ovadiah Yoseph, the former Sefaradic Chief Rabbi of Israel, has suggested that, in reaction to this shift in societal norms, rabbis might once again revert to treating suicides according to the strict letter of the law.

I would now like turn our attention to euthanasia itself. It is important to point out that the definition of the term and the aim of the practice is a "good death," and only one person is dying—the patient. In this discussion the focus should be primarily on the individual, not on the family, not on the physician, not on the hospital administrator, not on the minister of health nor on the budget director.

In this sensitive and difficult area, there are significant differences of opinion even among accepted Orthodox halakhic authorities, because the interpretation of the basic texts and their degree of relevance to modern dilemmas is not easy and rarely straightforward. Therefore individuals of great erudition, scholarship, and conscience may interpret the same texts differently.

The spectrum of possibilities for euthanasia begins with active euthanasia, which, of course, may be involuntary (against the wishes of the patient), nonvoluntary, or voluntary. None of these are sanctioned by the Torah, no matter how difficult the circumstances. The command not to take human life continues to be valid, and there is unanimity on this point. With respect to active euthanasia, it makes little difference whether the patient has only a few minutes or a few years to live—active, purposeful taking of life is a capital crime in Judaism.

The Shulkhan Arukh goes so far as to forbid the moving, or even the touching, of the person who is in the death throes, for fear of hastening his death, even by a few moments. The picturesque example given compares the dying person to a flickering candle—any movement may extinguish the flame. Similarly, any untoward movement of the patient may be the final push from life over to death—a forbidden act.

Is our tradition callous to the suffering of the patient? Do our rabbis really feel that there are no situations perhaps even worse than death? No, indeed we do recognize that in certain situations continued suffering may be a fate worse than death. There is little glorification of suffering in the Jewish tradition. And there are several sources which may be interpreted to permit, and even perhaps encourage, prayer to the Almighty for the death of a suffering patient.

One of the most moving and dramatic stories describes the terminal illness and death of Rabbi Judah the Prince. [7] His rabbinic colleagues and students decreed a public fast and prayed for his recovery, as did his maid, known for her wisdom. But when she observed the degree of her master's suffering and the indignity to which he was subjected by his unrelenting diarrhea, she decided that it was more appropriate to pray for his death. But her prayers stood no chance against those of the great rabbis, who continued in their pleas for his recovery. The Talmud describes graphically and movingly a dramatic heavenly struggle between those on earth who wanted Rabbi Judah's recovery and the angels in heaven who were beckoning him to heaven. In desperation, and with great ingenuity, it is told that Rabbi Judah's maid threw a pitcher on the ground. The noise distracted the rabbis from their prayer, and, with this impediment to death removed, the tide turned in favor of the maid's prayers, and Rabbi Judah's soul departed in peace.

The Talmud seems to have approved of this simple woman's act, although some authorities note that the rabbinical contemporaries of Rabbi Judah acted differently than the maid, and perhaps it is their view that should prevail. There are several other references in Jewish sources which seem to legitimize the prayer for death.

But the permission to pray for the death of a suffering patient was limited by an extraordinarily perceptive, and currently most relevant, insight by a nineteenth century Turkish rabbi, Haim Palache. [8] He was approached by a pious member of his community who was in a serious ethical quandary. His wife had been seriously ill and suffering for many years with an incurable illness. Her suffering had now reached a point where she no longer could tolerate her distress. Euthanasia was clearly out of the question for this pious Jew and his wife. But he asked the rabbi whether or not he was permitted to pray for his wife's death, since recovery was essentially impossible. Rabbi Palache, in a sensitive and meticulous review of the relevant Jewish sources, concluded that indeed there were grounds to permit such prayer when suffering is so great that death may properly be seen as a deliverance much to be desired. But he added a critical limitation, that only those who have no involvement in the care of the patient may pray for the patient's death, because only they can do so objectively. But family members, or members of the health care team, who are burdened in any way by the responsibility of the care of the patient, may not pray for the patient's death, since their prayer may be tainted with a degree of self-interest. The Jewish tradition is extraordinarily sensitive to the subtle biases that may influence life and death decisions, even in the best-motivated and pious individuals. The relevance of this insight in our era of managed care and "bottom line" considerations is obvious.

What about what has been referred to as passive euthanasia, i.e., withholding therapy which may be life prolonging in order to shorten life? There are philosophers who contend that there is no ethical difference between passive and active euthanasia. In general, these philosophers are not contending that just as one forbids active euthanasia so too one should forbid passive euthanasia. On the contrary, almost invariably they are trying to convince those who do not treat everyone maximally that by the same logic they should not hesitate to perform active euthanasia.

I find it fascinating to note that physicians, nurses, and other individuals who personally deliver care for the patients, and who are the ones whose actions determine whether a patient shall live or die, as well as when and how the individual will die, often reject the philosophers' equation of active and passive euthanasia. Their intuitive response is that there is a difference between active killing and merely withholding a therapeutic act. And I believe that ethicists and philosopers would do well not to reject such intuitive responses out of hand. The *halakhah* too backs this intuitive response and posits an unequivocal difference between an act of omission and one of commission, with respect to culpability.

Having made this point, I prefer to avoid altogether the use of the term "passive euthanasia," even for those acts of omission which the *halakhah* might sanction. The goal should not be the death of the patient. The goal should be the avoidance of suffering and the elimination of barriers to the natural process of death, not the hastening of death. One may argue that this represents quibbling over semantics, but I believe that terminology is important medically, philosophically, and emotionally.

The Jewish tradition recognizes the permissibility of removing a factor that prevents the death of a dying patient. There are two unusual examples cited in the Shulkhan Arukh which describe a patient in the throes of death (*goses*) whose imminent death seems delayed by one of two stimuli, one was noise created by a woodchopper near the patient, or salt on the tongue of the patient. Either of these phenomena, perceived as impediments to the death of the patient, may be removed because such removal is not considered active termination of life but merely removal of obstacles to the departure of the soul.

Another example cited in support of the permissibility of removal of impediments to death is the moving description of the martyrology of Rabbi Hanina ben Tradyon. [9] When he was immolated by the Romans, they placed layers of wet wool on his chest to prolong his suffering. When the rabbi's students witnessed the suffering of their rabbi, they suggested that he inhale the flames to hasten his death, to which he replied: "Better that the Lord who gave me my life take it from me rather than that I should contribute to my demise." While the Roman executioner witnessed the scene, he too apparently was moved, and he asked the rabbi whether he might attain a place in heaven if he hastened the rabbi's death. The rabbi replied in the affirmative, whereupon the executioner raised the flames, removed the wool, and then in a final act of personal repentance leaped into the flames and perished together with Rabbi Hanina. At this point, a heavenly voice proclaimed that both Rabbi Hanina and the executioner entered heaven.

It is not easy to translate any of these examples into modern idiom. What are the modern analogies of the woodchopper, the salt, or the removal of the wet wool? There are significant differences of opinion among established halakhic experts on each of these points.

Individual, seemingly similar, cases may be different enough in subtle but important ways, so as to yield different conclusions. It is therefore not easy to derive generalizable rules. For example: how does one define a dying patient, a *goses*? The classic definition is that of a patient expected to die within seventy-two hours, but there is considerable controversy as to the exact definition. Some experts have even stated that we simply do not know. Prediction of death is at best a very inexact science, even by the experts in intensive care whose professional life is spent treating critically ill patients, as Dr. Joanne Lynn and her colleagues have so convincingly shown over the past few years. [10] When dealing with a patient who has been judged to be incurable, that is, the basic illness is no longer amenable to specific treatment and who is suffering, most Jewish authorities agree that the patient may refuse obtrusive, complex, and distressing treatments, which may be regarded not as life saving, but rather as merely prolonging the death process.

Those treatments, which many feel may be refused, include dialysis, attachment to a respirator, resuscitation, surgery, chemotherapy, and the like. On the other hand, straightforward, safe, simple treatments, such as antibiotics for an intercurrent infection or a blood transfusion for severe anemia, should be given. Feeding and fluids by mouth should certainly not be withheld, nor should simple intravenous fluids to prevent dehydration. Most authorities would also not permit withdrawal of tube feeding, although if a patient would have to be restrained in order to insert a feeding tube, such force-feeding would not be mandated by all authorities.

It cannot be overemphasized that pain relief must be offered in quantities sufficient to relieve suffering, even if such treatment shortens life. Actually more and more data are accumulating, suggesting that adequate and humane pain relief may not only not shorten life, but may prolong life. The treatment of pain still leaves much to be desired in even the best Western hospitals because of ignorance and/or callousness.

What roles do the patients' wishes have in these decisions? Here indeed there seems to be a clear acceptance of, and respect for, the patients' desires by most halakhic authorities. While theoretically a Jewish court (*bet din*) may compel therapy on an unwilling patient, in the real world today no such authority exists. In practice most authorities do not favor actual physical coercion to treatment. When one is dealing with a dying patient who is suffering, one should accept the patient's refusal of those treatments which he/she regards as without adequate benefit/cost ratio for himself/herself.

Most halakhic authorities do differentiate between withdrawal of therapy already begun and withholding of therapy, although many philosophers and physicians regard the two processes as ethically identical. The *halakhah* is particularly strict when withdrawal of a therapy such as disconnection of a respirator is followed immediately by death. But there are valid halakhic ways in special circumstances for terminating therapy without a direct causation of death.

I would caution again that it is difficult to give precise guidelines for individual cases. There are often subtle differences between seemingly identical cases which may result in opposite halakhic rulings. There is also as yet no unanimity of opinion in each situation. The field is dynamic; new and difficult dilemmas are being posed daily, and new specific decisions often carve out new ground and new precedents. We are, after all, dealing with life and death matters.

It is critical to emphasize that a great deal of objectivity is essential in these decisions. The only concern of the *halakhah* is the welfare of the patient under discussion. It is clear when one reads much of the general literature on the subject that all too often it is the interests of the family, the staff, and/ or the society that may influence the decision, usually in a direction of terminating the patient's life. These considerations are totally unacceptable by our tradition.

One of the unfortunate effects of the almost universal transfer of the locale of death to the hospital and even more so into the intensive care unit is the conversion of a natural process into a battlefield environment. And just like modern warfare is dominated by technology, so too is today's dying scene. Some of the undesirable consequences of this change are:

1. the fostering of the illusion that death is conquerable—if but we make the effort,

2. the loss of the critical emotional and social support by family and friends in the death process, and

3. the deprivation of the ultimate equanimity and resolution of life issues on the part of the patient.

In times gone by, the confession (*vidui*) by the dying person was an integral part of the Jewish dying process. While not a *sine qua non* for status in the world to come, as last rites may be for the Roman Catholic, the confession nevertheless was an important and standard procedure for a seriously ill person. With what I call the Americanization of the death process even among pious Jews, there has been a marked reduction in the undertaking of this religiously and psychologically therapeutic step of squaring accounts with one's maker and one's family before death and then being able to accept death's inevitability as a natural finale to a life well lived.

I would like to close with a bit of a digression from the Jewish view on life and death, to the Jewish view on another subject which bears on the present discussion.

A few months ago I received a letter from a prominent secular philosopher ethicist who is doing some research on the slippery slope concept, and he asked me whether there are traditional Jewish sources that address the issue. Indeed there are. There is a clear acknowledgment of human nature in its ability to rationalize and to blur distinctions, if it so suits the individual and the society's purpose. I believe that in the field of treatment of the terminally ill and euthanasia the rapidly changing societal attitudinal changes that have taken place over the past two decades are clear evidence that the slopes are indeed slippery. While unquestionably the overuse of life-sustaining technologies and the arrogant paternalism of physicians have contributed in a major way to changing attitudes, it is hard to escape the conclusion that these objective realities do not explain fully the course of events.

The Dutch experience is particularly troubling. Although only a few short years ago we were repeatedly and emphatically assured that the safeguards, as originally proposed, would prevent any abuses, the reality has proven otherwise. Thousands of cases of nonvoluntary euthanasia of adults and children have taken place, and further erosions are on the horizon. As one Dutch physician told me recently when he was asked how it felt to actively kill a patient, "The first time was difficult." Subsequent cases were much easier for him. So too it seems that each step along the path towards societally encouraged active euthanasia is a natural progression from the previous one.

I believe firmly that it would be a tragic mistake to join the stampede toward changing our Jewish medical tradition, which has been a beacon of humanity and sensitivity towards human life and human suffering.

NOTES

1. Tractate Sanhedrin, *Babylonian Talmud,* 4: 5.
2. Tractate Avot, *Babylonian Talmud,* 4: 22.
3. Tractate Shabbat, *Babylonian Talmud,* 151b.
4. Baruch Brody, *Life and Death Decision Making* (New York: Oxford University Press, 1988.)
5. Leviticus 19:16.
6. Deuteronomy 22:2.
7. Tractate Ketubot, *Babylonian Talmud,* 104a.
8. Haim Palache, *Hikekei Lev.,* vol.1, responsum 50, (Salonika Book Export Enterprises, Ltd., 1840; 1978).
9. Tractate Avodah Zarah, *Babylonian Talmud,* 18a.
10. William Knaus, D.P. Wagner, Joanne Lynn, "Short-Term Mortality Predictions for Critically Ill Hospitalized Adults: Science and Ethics," *Science* 254 (1991): 389–94.

The Sanctity-of-Human-Life Doctrine

DAVID C. THOMASMA, PH.D.

The sanctity of human life as a doctrine or assumed value in medicine has been both neglected and overstated in the past twenty-five years. The neglect of the doctrine takes the form of unexamined and unreflective appeals to the "sanctity of human life" as a background for ethical analysis of medicine. The overstatements arise from the increasingly shrill, equally unexamined, assertions of some more extreme pro-life advocates and unsupported attestations of religious traditions. Both the neglect and the overstatements have contributed to a new examination of the doctrine in post-modern bioethical thought. So far that reexamination has proven detrimental to the meaning and recognition of the doctrine and its importance for bioethics.

In this essay I shall lay out briefly the history of the doctrine and its importance for medicine and bioethics, the recent condemnations of the doctrine and the reasons for those condemnations, and the possible reconstruction of the meaning of the doctrine in modern bioethics.

THE SANCTITY-OF-HUMAN-LIFE DOCTRINE

The reason that the "sanctity of human life" is referred to as a "doctrine" lies in its origins in the Judeo-Christian tradition. It is a religious teaching.

THE JEWISH TRADITION

The first experience of Yahweh in human history was of an intervening and saving God, capable of directing the chosen people and their fortunes, first in the centuries of wandering in the desert, later in their captivity in Egypt, their salvation from that slavery (the Exodus), and their claiming the land of Judea for their own. Throughout this several-thousand-year history, Yahweh was worshiped as the one God that chose his people through original and renewed covenants. Hence the notion of the intrinsic dignity of human life, although only incipient at this time, is closely tied to God's choice of a people he wills to call his own. This "specialness" extends only to the chosen tribes, and not to their enemies. Holy war is possible and even seems to be demanded by the saving God in order to bring down false gods and peoples who would destroy his chosen race.

Gradually, as the covenants are renewed and the kingdom is established with its Temple worship, Jewish thought broadened the implications of the covenant to include the notion that the "chosen people" by that very choice were a "holy people," dedicated, just like the priestly caste, to the honor and glory of God. Once again this holiness, an expression of intrinsic human dignity or "sanctity," stemmed from God's choice of them to be his witnesses in human history, not from their creation by him. Indeed, the notion of a "creator God" did not seem to appear until after the destruction of the Temple and the exile in Babylon.

One might be tempted to think that this notion of a creator God occurred to the Jewish people in conjunction with their integration into Babylonian society and its influence on their thinking. Certainly this influence is present. Yet it actually appears from a salvation experience again. Recall the Psalm (137:1–4): "There by the rivers of Babylon, we hung up our harps. There we sat and wept. . . . How can we worship God in a foreign land?"— an exile lament. With the destruction of the Temple, and the loss of the Ark of the Covenant along with the corresponding daily sacrifice to Yahweh, the Israelites were forced to reconfigure and reinterpret their faith. The exile itself was an eye-opening experience for them, during which they discovered that they could remain faithful to their God outside their own territory or "place." Their God was not confined, like other gods around the known world, to a specific place. This was part of their salvation history. After all, he led them out of Egypt into the Promised Land. God was an all-over God. Thence, from their own salvation history, the Jewish people began to see that God not only saved them, but was also master of human and natural history, the creator of the universe and of all lands and peoples. This recognition, displayed clearly in the creation accounts of the first chapter of Genesis, comes from both a then-current scientific understanding of creation and a faith history that is developed by the post-exilic priestly tradition centered in the restored Temple in Jerusalem.

Insofar as the "sanctity of human life" arose from this religious tradition, it is essential to realize its primary origin in salvation history and only secondary origin in a theory of creation. I will come back to this point in later analysis.

THE CHRISTIAN TRADITION

Christianity arose as a branch of Judaism and continued this tradition of viewing God as both saving and redeeming human beings who, on their own, were not capable of rescuing themselves from sin. Yet it broadened the notion of the chosen people to include all human beings who were both called by God to be "grafted on" to the root of Jesse (to use St. Paul's metaphor) and were redeemed from their sinfulness by the sacrifice of the unblemished Jesus Christ on the cross, who died "once for all." As an exemplar and in his teaching, Jesus demonstrated effectively the dignity of others, even those who accused him and harmed him, through his nonviolent responses. This lack of vindication, this seeming abstention from the ancient rule of an "eye for an eye and a tooth for a tooth," had a tremendous impact not only on Jesus' early followers, but throughout the course of Western civilization.

The early Christian church was largely pacificist. [1] Nonetheless, it contained within it the seeds of ambiguity about those whose professions might lead them to kill or execute others. Military members, civil officials, and judges were welcomed into the community without explicit requirements that they abandon their profession. Nevertheless, killing and suicide are prohibited in the Scriptures, the Didache, and other early documents and writings. This belief can be contrasted with the pre-Christian era. In ancient times only the Buddhists adopted an official nonviolent attitude toward the world. All other religions, including Judaism in the Old Testament, regarded war and killing as a necessary evil.

Jesus was a social critic and an agitator. [2] This is why he was crucified. The context of his ministry included both nonviolent sit-ins by Jewish citizens against Roman authorities (for desecrating the Temple and hoisting graven images) [3] as well as violent resistance by a largely Galilean group called "the Zealots." In contrast to his fellow Galileans, Jesus advocated nonviolence, love of enemies, doing good to those who persecute, turning the other cheek. On the other hand, Jesus himself violently drove out the money changers from the Temple, calling them thieves who desecrated his Father's house. He accepted the Roman centurion's (a soldier's) faith in his power to heal the centurion's servant boy, yet told Peter to put away his sword because "Those that live by the sword, die by the sword."

This ambivalence, at least according to one method of interpreting the Christian tradition, is an essential feature of imitating Jesus that is required of Christians, "to take up the cross and follow him." [4] As Yoder argues from this perspective:

The believer's cross is no longer any and every kind of suffering, sickness, or tension, the bearing of which is demanded. The believer's cross must be, like his Lord's, the price of his social nonconformity. It is not, like sickness or catastrophe, an inexplicable, unpredictable suffering; it is the end of a path freely chosen after counting the cost. [5]

Accordingly, the main temptation of Jesus in the Scriptures seems to have been, like all good Jews around him, to counteract the Roman dominion of the Holy Land and their desecration of Jewish law by exercising social responsibility "in the interest of justified revolution, through the use of available violent methods." [6] The fact that he did not succumb to this temptation, but chose nonviolence, was not lost on his followers. They understood that the Reign of God preached by Jesus was a new social order of love and that challenging violence by their own nonresistance in imitation of Jesus, they would be persecuted and put to death by secular powers for taking a stand against socially accepted violence. [7] Further to the point of this essay, the fundamental reason for this social order that included the requirement of love for all persons, friends and enemies alike, was that God is Love, and that all humans are created and redeemed by him. This point is stated and restated continuously in the New Testament. Here are two examples:

> If you love only those who love you, what credit is that to you . . . ? But you must love your enemies, and do good and lend without expecting return . . . you will be sons of the Most High, because he himself is kind to the ungrateful and wicked. Be compassionate as your Father is compassionate. [8]
>
> Love your enemies and pray for your persecutors; only so can you be children of your heavenly Father who makes his sun rise on good and bad alike, and sends the rain on the honest and dishonest. . . . You must therefore be all goodness, just as your heavenly Father is all good. [9]

As noted, the early church, while condemning participating in killing, accepted as members converts who included military personnel, civic officials, and judges—persons who might be expected to kill or execute in fulfillment of their duties. Further, since the early Christians were a tiny minority of the population, they did not have to worry about being subsumed into the political power structures and could maintain the creative tension over and against society that marked their self-understanding. There is evidence that conscientious objection was a continuous Christian response to the state. Celsus complained around A.D. 180 that if all men were Christians the empire would become prey to barbarians, and Origen's answer to Celsus seventy years later demonstrates continued commitment to nonviolence. [10] The first three centuries were therefore marked by conscientious objection from a substantial number of Christians, and a willingness to die rather than acknowledge a supposed divinity of the emperor.

But by the time Christianity became the official religion of the Roman Empire, referred to as the Constantinian Church due to the influence of Constantine's conversion, the church had to grapple with the complex problem of now being counted among the "principalities and powers" of the world. It gradually had to accommodate to secular society and establish norms to govern its responses to new challenges about which Jesus or the tradition said nothing. As Martin notes:

> The period from the apostolic age to the age of Constantine was one in which Christianity developed from a Jewish sect into the heir of Roman civilization. As it did so the Church assimilated alien influences, such as the philosophy of the Stoics, which assisted it in the formulation of norms which should regulate its relation to society. The attempts to find such norms and the compromises [entailed] inevitably brought the question of the Church and its attitude to war into focus. [11]

The Christian community gradually accommodated itself to secular society since it gained an official role therein, and the habit of relying upon different secular philosophies and movements to strengthen its standing in and against contemporary mores continued throughout its history. At the time of Constantine and thereafter officials and soldiers of the state had to be given more explicit guidelines about the rule against killing. The accommodation to secular society eventually took the form of permitting certain forms of killing under very strict, exceptional circumstances (such as the conditions articulated for a just war). The rule against killing was paramount in its definition of the limits of personal dominion over the lives of others and oneself. It was then and still is today a form of respecting both the inherent dignity of human lives and the divinity of a universal God.

Essentially, the rule against killing is a form of faith in God himself, a faith that God who created and redeemed can also save those whom he will. The prophetic tradition of the Old Testament emphasized that God would fight for his people of faith: "Not by might, nor by power, but by my Spirit, says Yahweh of Hosts" [12] and "He will guard the feet of his faithful ones; for not by might shall a man prevail." [13] This salvation theme was underscored in limiting the use of violence and death in civil society through the rule against killing.

In the Middle Ages, those who used the sword or knife in a previous profession (soldiers or surgeons) were considered to have a canonical impediment for the priesthood. [14] Even during the Inquisition, an acknowleged low point in the church's history, the condemned were turned over to secular authorities for the carrying out of their sentence of death. There was in this action an incipient "separation" of church and state, though their goals were similar. As history has shown, the sanctity-of-human-life doctrine has suffered the most when religion is suppressed or subsumed into social policy. The Holocaust is the most obvious example.

Throughout the church's history, groups or orders within it testified to the creative tension vis-à-vis the world, but the church as a whole continued to embrace a number of different and potentially discordant positions. Protestant scholars call this the "Catholic compromise" and argue that this compromise with secular society led to the need for the Reformation. [15] During and after the Reformation, a number of sects of Christians arose that developed further the nonviolence of Jesus as a centerpiece of their churches. Among these were the Mennonites, Quakers, and Church of the Brethren. Each of their nonviolent positions was derived slightly differently from the Bible, but all rested on the sanctity of human life. [16]

THE SANCTITY OF LIFE AND BIOETHICS

As can be gleaned from this brief recounting of the development of the doctrine of sanctity of life, it can mean many things, different things, even opposed things to different persons or groups who appeal to it. Let us briefly consider some of the major categories of meaning the doctrine assumes within the sphere of bioethics today.

VITALISM

The first category includes all meanings that appeal to the notion, developed above, that human beings are created and redeemed by God and share in some mysterious way, through that creation and redemption, in God's holiness. Thus the "sanctity" of human life means just that, that the physical as well as the historical lives of human beings are filled with God's holy presence.

According to this interpretation, one must respect all forms of human life from conception to death as being redeemed and grace-filled. Even if one cannot prove that some forms of human life are derivative, now decayed, or even wholly personal, that does not exempt one from respecting that life as holy. Hence one cannot deliberately destroy any form of human life (as one might be able to destroy an animal's life, since it is created but not "redeemed" by God). This would include embryos, fetuses, the retarded, the neurologically impaired, and the dying. To respect the value or sanctity of human life would be equivalent in this interpretation to respecting God, since any human life, regardless of its status, includes some of the holiness of God.

This position in bioethics is often called "vitalism," since it extends to human life some of the absolute qualities of the divine. One finds it employed most often at the bedside of the dying patient. Sometimes vitalism is taken in an absolute sense, such that no treatment or intervention can be withdrawn from the patient because to do so would show disrespect to God's own power and life within that person. At other times, vitalism is relativized by the balance between the effort (burdens) and benefits (outcomes) for the patient. When the burdens become too high relative to benefits, then proper respect for the sanctity of life is to let go of our human interventions and let God call the person to himself. Note that this analysis maintains respect for the sanctity of human life. Autonomy, or self-determination, has little place in this approach, since one is required to take proper care of one's life that has come as a gift from God, and one is therefore not completely free to manage or control one's destiny.

Ironically, some interpretations within this tradition distinguish between personal and nonpersonal forms of human life, such that abortion might be recognized as legitimate in some circumstances but not withdrawal of life-support at the end of life. In effect, these various interpretations are still vitalist, as they share the notion of human life as an absolute value, but ascribe such life only to specific forms of human life that are obviously personal. As in all extreme positions, the opposites meet: one might find very conservative Orthodox Jews and pro-life Christians in this interpretative position along with very liberal and committed pacifists.

CONSISTENT ETHIC OF LIFE

A different, nonvitalist, interpretation of the sanctity-of-life doctrine has sprung up in the Catholic tradition. It is called "the consistent ethic of life" and was championed by, among others, the late Joseph Cardinal Bernardin of Chicago. A look at the earlier pronouncements of popes about bioethical issues bears witness to the impact of this view as well. [17] "The consistent ethic of life," or what is known popularly as the "seamless garment" argument [18] cuts across all forms of denigration, from rejection of abortion to euthanasia, but also from unjust war to capital punishment, and from discrimination against the vulnerable to the oppression of the poor, the elderly, and the homeless. Despite the American Catholic bishops' condemnation of nuclear warfare and capital punishment in line with that consistent ethic of life, along with similar and parallel condemnations by other Christian bodies, these violations of the rule against killing do not provoke the same sense of moral outrage among my fellow churchgoers as euthanasia does. I find this especially odd, since among all forms of killing, the least objectionable would seem to be that which is done at the repeated request of the one who suffers, with the motive to relieve that suffering, and in the presence of the inevitability of death.

Further, the religious argument against euthanasia and assisted suicide is the only one that might make sense, since as has been shown, the philosophical, legal, and professional arguments for and against euthanasia and assisted suicide seem to balance each other out. [19, 20] As social acceptance of the practice of assisting death becomes more widespread, and its legal status is gradually clarified, it seems appropriate to look at the question of the sanctity of life from a much richer background than that of ethical analysis alone.

The nonvitalist but life-committed viewpoint goes like this. All forms of human life are created and redeemed by God. This means that we must honor all forms of human life in every circumstance, from conception to death. To be "consistent" means that one cannot profess the sanctity of human life before birth and then neglect the social circumstances of human beings once born. Yet this does not mean that human beings are in themselves "divine." There is an enormous divide between God and his creatures. To be human is not to be divine, but only to share in that divinity through God's grace. Again to use a New Testament metaphor from St. Paul, God has adopted human beings into his own household, as members of his family.

Instead of a vitalist interpretation, then, each form of human life is considered to be "innocent" and worthy of respect across the board, until a willful act creates a loss of innocence, say by becoming an unjust aggressor against others through murder or warfare. Then that person loses the right to his or her life under strict conditions established, for example, in Just War Theory, the rigid guidelines and appeals structure of capital punishment, or the warnings that the police must first issue before firing a gun in pursuit of a perpetrator.

Within this view of the sanctity of human life, one cannot justify the manipulation of frozen embryos, abortion of fetuses, [21] or assisting in suicide or euthanasia, on the grounds that one would be violating the intrinsic value of innocent human life. Yet one might be justified, although this is also problematic at present, in the taking of certain specific, publically processed and declared noninnocent human lives. For most within this tradition, the right to take noninnocent human life is upheld, but the practical realities of determining such procedures that can be upheld in justice are difficult and may no longer apply in today's violent world. It was certainly the case that Cardinal Bernardin condemned nuclear warfare and capital punishment as do all American Catholic bishops.

In effect, this particular interpretation of the sanctity-of-human-life doctrine creates a *prima facie* duty to respect all forms of human life because they are created and redeemed by God, but does not rule out the formalized process of determining when other values might override such duties, values such as defense of one's country or property, or public punishment for murder and social mayhem. More important for bioethics, this nonvitalist position signifies that, although human life is intrinsically valuable, it is not an absolute value. One must balance respect for the value of human life with other values, particularly at its end, when burdensome efforts to prolong life can be withheld and withdrawn. These actions are nevertheless considered respectful since they respect the created and limited meaning of human life by not transposing one's gaze from the ultimate source of its meaning in God. Greater weight is given than in the vitalist position to human self-determination about the point at which burdens would outweigh benefits through advance or current directives to this effect.

RESPECT FOR HUMAN LIFE

A third position in the sanctity-of-life constellation is held by many who do not share the belief systems of organized religion, but wish to uphold the intrinsic value of human life. Largely philosophically based, this position extracts a rationalist or essentialist view from the religious connotations. In essence it holds that human life has special provenance compared with other life forms like animals and the environment. Thus, the "sanctity" of human life comes to mean the primacy of place for human life in the value hierarchy of duties. In this interpretation, too, human life can be both intrinsically and extrinsically valued.

Since the values attached to human life can be both intrinsic and extrinsic, a balance between the values can sometimes tilt from intrinsic value towards extrinsic. Thus, persons holding this tradition of bioethical analysis have little difficulty in justifying the preponderance of value for a mother's choice to abort a fetus because she is farther along the scale of personal and moral development than is a fetus, and has a constellation of both intrinsic and extrinsic values, duties, responsibilities, etc. that is unmatched by the fetus. Similarly, one could possibly justify removing life support from a person in a permanent vegetative state or coma because their intrinsic value as persons is now reduced to their biography and their extrinsic value to others becomes more objectified. This position bleeds into the following one.

THE VALUE OF HUMAN LIFE

According to this category of the sanctity-of-life doctrine, human life has a value, but is not necessarily always intrinsically valued. Interpreters in this category see the doctrine as defining human life vis-à-vis other animal lives. For the most part, human life takes precedence over other types of life and even the environment, but not always. Proponents might argue that a healthy orangutan cannot be killed to harvest a heart for a diseased infant, for example. This is because the risk and likely outcomes for the infant are not sufficient to endanger the healthy life of another living being. [22] One might imagine that ethicists in this category could acknowledge the created nature of the infant (as well as the orangutan) without it impelling them to justify ranking the infant in her condition higher than the orangutan in its healthier one.

Further, certain forms of human life can be extrinsically valued, i.e., be objectively valued, since there is little or no consciousness, e.g., embryos, early fetuses, the severely cognitively impaired, and the like. Thus, when either premature or impaired developmentally, some forms of human life can be valued for their importance to others within a family or society itself, and not for their own sakes. One could then argue that abortion is justified, since the fetus is less developmentally able than a conscious adult in a moral quandary. Or one could argue that the only value of an unconscious, dying patient, is to her family. One is justified in taking her life at her request unless there is some overriding need of family to keep her alive for a few days. Her intrinsic value, then, was tagged to her personhood that has now vanished, leaving an empty shell of a body kept alive by medical technology. Indeed, true respect is centered on her former condition of life and can now only be salvaged by obeying her wishes to die.

The same reasoning would also apply to those who support research on embryos or using fetal tissue for transplants to help people with diabetes, Alzheimer's, or macular degeneration. In the latter instance, fetal tissue transplants, the sanctity-of-human-life argument takes the form of a utilitarian notion that greater good can come from the tragedy of abortion (about which the researchers or doctors had nothing to do) by benefitting others. Thus, Mark Siegler, commenting on the first macular degeneration fetal tissue transplant surgery which took place at his institution, said that this "should not be viewed as an endorsement of abortion which remains a tragic situation, but rather an effort to treat a previously incurable disease." [23] Those who hold a more rigorous view of the sanctity of human life predictably condemned the procedure. The Roman Catholic Archdiocese of Chicago said that using cells from an unborn child "can only be viewed as an endorsement of abortion, which many in our country find ethically unacceptable. A good end can never justify an immoral means." The strict pro-life position on the surgery was reflected by Ann Scheidler who said that the surgery was "reminiscent of the Nazi experiments on human beings." [24]

It should be noted, however, that all three of these positions stem from a respectful notion of the value of the fetus' life. That is why I included Siegler's position in that tradition. There are many bioethicists who do not agonize about the value of a fetus' life and have no difficulty whatsoever in justifying the use of fetal tissue to help others. In fact, some of them even endorse the creation of research embryos who would be destroyed after the research is completed prior to cell differentiation at about fourteen days.

THE PRESERVATION OF LIFE

Finally, the sanctity of human life can be a shorthand phrase in medicine and in bioethics for the goal of medicine. This goal is traditionally seen as the "preservation of human life." By appealing to the sanctity of human life, one attempts to make it a primary and unquestioned principle of medicine such that to ignore or desecrate it would be to violate the fundamental nature of medicine itself.

A very profound version of this view was articulated by Leon Kass, who argues that at the end of life, humanity is owed to the dying, not humaneness. By this he means that compassion for animals who cannot make decisions for themselves and are in our complete dominion requires our humaneness in euthanizing them so that they no longer suffer. This act, however, is inappropriate for human beings who possess a different set of rights and duties stemming from their own humanity. [25] For them only our own personal outreach and compassion will suffice. Kass is committed to the preservation of human life based on its intrinsic value. Speaking of euthanasia, Kass says:

> People who care for autonomy and dignity should try to reverse this dehumanization of the last stages of life, instead of giving dehumanization its final triumph by welcoming the desperate good-bye-to-all that is contained in one final plea for poison. [26]

THE DOCTRINE TODAY

There was, until recently, only theoretical interest in the metaphysical problem of personhood and its intrinsic value, except perhaps in ancient times in arguments about the unity of God in three persons, or more contemporaneously over problems of slavery and racism. In the final analysis, Plato's, Aristotle's, Hume's, Locke's, Descartes' positions on personhood formerly did not make a big impact on everyday decisions. [27] However, the broad applicability and popularity of bioethics issues demonstrate the importance of principles that relate directly to practical and public policy actions such as abortion, research on embryos, the discontinuance of feeding tubes from severely affected stroke victims, or physician-assisted suicide and euthanasia. The sanctity-of-human-life doctrine plays such a central role in bioethics.

The contemporary attack on the sanctity-of-human-life doctrine is characterized by a failure to distinguish among the different forms of meaning the doctrine takes. Which interpretation is one arguing against? I take up antivitalism, rationalism, and pluralism as three current movements around the sanctity-of-human-life question.

ANTIVITALISM

Some objections to the sanctity-of-life doctrine are formulated on the basis of a balance of duties to human life beyond that of simply preserving life. In essence this represents an objection to the vitalist interpretation of sanctity of life. Excellent examples of this philosophical analysis are provided by Daniel Callahan and Baruch Brody in their respective discussions of abortion. Callahan argued philosophically that one cannot deduce that no taking of life is possible from the sanctity-of-life doctrine alone. In his words,

> A major objection worth leveling at any rigidly restrictive moral code on abortion is that it is prone to hold that an absolute prohibition of induced abortion is a logical entailment of "the sanctity of human life." The logical route leading to this prohibition is that "the sanctity of life" means and can only mean under all circumstances that bodily life is to be preserved, which in turn is taken to entail a prohibition of the taking of fetal life. No room is left, in this deductive chain, for a recognition of other demands of the principle. [28]

For his part, Brody developed an essentialist argument against abortion. The lines of his philosophical argument are that once a fetus is determined to be a form of human life, there are only two legitimate conditions under which its life could be taken to save another human life, and these occur so rarely that they could hardly justify the current social policy. Only one condition applies to abortion in any event. He says of Callahan's argument:

> ... Callahan's point, while quite right abstractly, sheds very little light on the issue of abortion. It remains for Callahan to suggest cases relevant to the issue of abortion in which this obligation not to take the life of a human being can be overridden. [29]

Brody notes that Callahan does give some examples, largely if and when society were so threatened as to lose its existence. As Brody notes, though, abandoning our social obligations to care for the helpless in times of emergency is not a good analogy with abortion since "it would certainly be incorrect to say that the communities in question took the lives of those helpless people." [30] Thus, one can agree that the obligation not to kill can sometimes be overridden by other obligations. These are very rare, and when they do occur, they more often than not take the form of protecting the sanctity of human life in society at the risk of harming individual lives, the common good taking precedence over individual good. One is hard-pressed to develop analogies to argue in favor of taking one life to save another. [31]

Both Brody and Callahan are nonvitalist adherents to the doctrine of the sanctity of human life. Their moorings in faith produce their philosophical analyses.

RATIONALISM

Modernity is also characterized by a loss of faith, by a loss of a sense of the meaning of life. A rational person examines all assumptions, including that of faith, and is pressured by reason and culture around him or her to abandon that faith for a more solid pathway of reason. This is called the "Enlightenment Project." A number of bioethicists have declared that the Enlightenment Project is dead and that a new path must be taken to provide a foundation for a moral life. [32] Often prominent thinkers turned away from reasoning to tackle the development of one's existence through time as the basis of the dignity of human life. There is a more remote connection than direct faith to the Creator and almost none to the Redeemer. As Tolstoy wrote about his own search for such a foundation for his life:

> There resulted in a contradiction, from which there were two ways out: either what I called rational was not so rational as I had thought;

or that which to me appeared irrational was not so irrational as I had thought. [33]

Tolstoy turned from book learning and academic pursuits towards cultivating a friendship with everyday persons. He gradually grew to love them and cherish them, and learning this love of life, he says, found the truth of its value. [34]

Along parallel lines Swenson argues that the sacredness and dignity of human life does not lie in a body of knowledge about life, but in the experience of the self as its comes to command its moral center. He calls this an "ethical view of life," and describes it as:

> ... the essence of life and its happiness is to be sought in the moral consciousness alone. ... This view holds that the individual human self has an infinite worth, that the personality has an eternal validity, that the bringing of this validity to expression in the manifold relations and complications of life is the true task of the self, that this task gives to the individual's historical development an infinite significance because it is a process through which the personality in its truth and depth comes to its own. [35]

It is not difficult to catch the connection of this existential and developmental account of the dignity of human life to one's ultimate good. It is described as a "tiny whisper" within the self, a good that should be seized as all else is relativized, a good that is one's ultimate meaning and truth in life. [36] Indeed, St. Thomas Aquinas called the constant yearning for happiness a "moral argument for the existence of God."

What we see under the rationalist tradition today is an abandonment and rejection of the objective natural law by which Enlightenment thinkers sought happiness in society under "Nature and Nature's god." The primary reason for rejecting this project is that so much of life is irrational, as Sartre demonstrated in his atheist works. Another reason is the awful experience of the scientific and technological civilization run amok in Germany during and in Russia after the Second World War. In choosing whether reason or unreason is a better path, like Tolstoy, one must turn to one's own development and promptings.

PLURALISM

Such an existential turn does not help in the end. Secular pluralism must be taken seriously. When it is, the argument goes, no single foundational belief system can predominate. Since there are so many competing versions of the moral life, one can only come to a moral decision through negotiation and compromise, while respecting peaceably each person and the community. [37] Compared to the religious tradition mapped out above, this is a very weak form of the sanctity-of-human-life doctrine, if a form of it at all. The reason persons are to be respected comes, not from their innate dignity or sacredness, but from the principle of tolerance for opposing viewpoints that is required by a peaceable society. [38]

Furthermore, a secular critique of the sanctity-of-life doctrine seems to undermine any residual meaning in application to current events and ethical issues. Traditional intellectual resources that have grounded medical theory and practice are commonly disparaged today as antiquated and quite irrelevant to high technology and entrepreneurial medicine. Peter Singer has explored the collapse of our traditional ethic, by which he means the traditional Judeo-Christian sanctity-of-life ethic. The demise was occasioned both by the increasing secularization of society and also by the demands of the new technology in medicine itself. Singer argues that rather than "patch up" the holes in the sanctity-of-life ethic that have appeared due to new technological challenges, it is far better to abandon this ethic altogether in favor of a more consistent clinical and public policy medical ethics. [39] As he says, "technological advances in medicine have made it impossible to retain the principle of the sanctity of human life." [40]

The basis of Singer's critique of the sanctity-of-life ethic is that it is inconsistent and confusing. Small wonder. What he presents is little more than a caricature. Statements he makes clearly fail to distinguish between the ethic derived from the doctrine, the different types enumerated above, and especially an almost deliberate, rhetorical effort to identify the sanctity-of-life doctrine with the most extreme forms of vitalism. He also characterizes pro-life and the Catholic tradition together as "unthinking," therefore explicitly suggesting that no right-thinking, rational human being could possibly adopt such positions. In fact, his description of the ethic fails on so many counts that it is nothing more than a "straw man." His assumption, critiqued by Callahan, posited as a universal, an uncompromising ethic that is guilty of duplicity, fictions (brain death), disguises, and convoluted reasoning (double effect) in order to avoid absolutism in practice, while paying lip service to the abstract principle of the uncompromisingly intrinsic value of human life. At its root, Singer's assumption that accepting the sanctity-of-life ethic commits one to vitalism is, as I have shown, false. There are other viable interpretations of the doctrine. In his final chapter, Singer enumerates a rational, autonomous, technological ethic for today's world, one that is coherent with all the assumptions of a modern, scientific society.

We are left with a contemporary version of the tension between religious faith and secular society that has perhaps eluded us since the Constantinian Church. Recall the view of Christianity that one acquires one's true freedom through suffering and not from avoiding that suffering. In suffering one seems to lose one's self, one's ultimate identity, one's autonomy. Applying this insight to suffering and death, Therese Lysaught rightly contends that "... rather than this loss of autonomy and self signaling the ultimate destruction of the person, it is in fact the condition for the constitution of true identity." [41] One can readily discern the opposition of this viewpoint with secular humanism like that of Bertrand Russell, [42] Albert Camus, [43] Julian Huxley, [44] and Richard Taylor, [45] to mention only a few, all of whom adopt a nontheistic response to the meaning of life. As a result, autonomy and self-determination are so predominant that those adopting the secular viewpoint in bioethics do not consider in their analyses of beginning and end-of-life decisions the obligation to care for life as a gift from God. [46,47] It is simply a nonfactor.

TOWARD A RECONSTRUCTION

It is clear that the attacks on the sanctity-of-life doctrine expose its vulnerability in a pluralistic society. Its religious origins are, as are the religious origins of all of Western civilization, increasingly called into question by secular critical thinkers. For one thing, such critical thinking frees us from the slavery of unquestioned or unexamined ideas, such as Socrates proclaimed, that the "unexamined life is not worth living." For those who still wish to cherish the value of human life, newer thinking and rethinking is required to answer the objections and to be persuasive about the importance of the doctrine and the dangers of abandoning it. As Colman McCarthy succinctly put it: "Whether expressed by Mother Teresa or Albert Schweitzer, reverence for life and the consistent honoring of that reverence is at the core of all life-or-death cases." [48]

One way of doing ethics today, in a pluralistic environment, is to forego the religious and metaphysical defense of important concepts like the sanctity of human life in favor of an experiential *a priori*. By this is meant that in the dialogue about values to be preserved in a pluralistic environment certain a prioris, or established truths, should be placed on the table as starting points. Experiential a prioris, unlike those purported to be grounded in metaphysical or religious truth, are instead based on the experience of our civilization, such as analogously, one might examine one's ethical options against the backdrop of one's own moral experience and conscience. Indeed, it is a mark of a wise and prudent individual to take cognizance of past experience, pitfalls, weaknesses, mistakes, and yes, even sins (willful harms to others and one's self), in contemplating a decision. A good example might be a person prone to anger who is cut off in traffic. He might contemplate how in the past he would speed up and make angry conversation and gestures through his open window at the other driver, to the detriment of his own safety and that of others. This time, he slows down instead, and lets the other driver annoy others up ahead.

Similarly, regarding bioethical and human life issues in medicine, we must analyze the past and place on the table some proposals for *a prioris* regarding the value of human life. Given the Holocaust, it is not a stretch to reflect that, in the absence of the belief about the instrinsic value of human life, medically technological civilization in the West tended to disvalue the neurologically vulnerable and poor, as well as the genetically "impure," to the point of active killing. If it had not happened in Germany, it would have happened somewhere else in the West, given our propensity to "solve" problems by objectifying the problem, breaking it into isolated and component parts, developing expertise for each isolated part, expertise itself isolated from common decision making, and commodifying the results of this expertise. In the midst of this propensity, it is too easy for our civilization to disvalue the whole of human life in favor of gaining ascendancy about our expertise regarding a part of it. A good example was the worry of scientists that, if we could not conduct research on human embryos, France might get ahead of the United States in this crucial area.

Without overstating this habit of mind, since it has many good consequences as well as bad ones, I would propose that the collective experience of Western civilization is that human life must be intrinsically valued. Otherwise, despite the good intentions of many alternate proposals, harms are introduced into the common good of human life. Thus, an experiential a priori for Western medicine must be what has been the sanctity-of-human-life doctrine.

CONCLUSION

I remain convinced that the experience of salvation, so overwhelming a gift from God, remains the primary conviction behind the sanctity-of-life doctrine, not the creation of individuals by God. Nonetheless, as I have shown in this essay, the doctrine itself is subject to a plethora of interpretations, even within broadly painted categories. The attacks on the doctrine today are not unexpected, given the multiplicity of interpretation and the vacuousness of appeals to the doctrine without serious reexamination of its meaning. My proposal for an experiential *a priori* respecting the intrinsic value of human life is only one possible avenue for reconstruction of the doctrine.

NOTES

1. The *New Catholic Encyclopedia* states that the early church was not clearly pacifist. The article analyzes the essential tension in Christian history between an abhorrence of social mayhem and following Christ's admonitions to respond nonviolently (see "Pacifism," *New Catholic Encyclopedia*, vol. 10 [New York: McGraw-Hill, 1967]: 855–57). Some Christian churches today adopt a wholly pacifist position (e.g., the Church of the Brethren, Mennonites), while pacifism is a position adopted by a minority in other mainstream churches. All share, however, in the conviction that human life is sacred or to be respected.

2. I trace the importance of this social criticism for the notion of the intrinsic value of human life in David C. Thomasma, *Human Life in the Balance* (Louisville, Ky.: Westminster Press, 1990): chap. 5.

3. Josephus, *Antiquities*, xviii.3. See also, Emil G. Kraeling, "The Episode of the Roman Standards at Jerusalem," *Harvard Theological Review* 35 (1942): 263ff.

4. This tradition is called "biblical" by which is meant that the biblical vision refuses to be pushed into any one single mold of current fashion or belief, but rather stands "in creative tension with the cultural functions of our age or perhaps of any age." John H.Yoder, *The Politics of Jesus* (Grand Rapids, Mich.: Eerdmans, 1972): 5.

5. Yoder, *The Politics of Jesus*, 97.

6. Yoder, *The Politics of Jesus*, 98.

7. Andre Trocmé, *Jésus-Christ et la révolution non-violente*, trans. Michael H. Shank and Martin E. Miller (Scottdale, Pa.: Herald Press, 1973): 124.

8. Luke 6:32–36 (AV)

9. Matthew 5:43–48 (NEB)

10. David A. Martin, *Pacifism: An Historical and Sociological Study* (London: Routledge & Kegan Paul, 1965): 33.

11. Martin, *Pacifism: An Historical and Sociological Study*, 33.

12. Zechariah 4:6.

13. 1 Samuel 2:9.

14. Such persons, called "conversi," or "converts," could become brothers in the orders, but not priests, even in such clerical orders as the Order of Friars Preachers (Dominicans). This impediment was present until the most recent revision of Canon Law after the Second Vatican Council.

15. Martin, *Pacifism: An Historical and Sociological Study*, 33.

16. Dale W. Brown, *Biblical Pacifism: A Peace Church Perspective* (Elgin, Ill.: Brethren Press, 1988).

17. E.g., Pius XI. Casti Canubii, Section 64. In William J. Gibbons, ed., *Seven Great Encyclicals* (Glen Rock, N.J.: Paulist Press, 1939): 95.

18. Joseph Cardinal Bernardin, *The Consistent Ethic of Life* (Kansas City, Mo.: Sheed and Ward, 1988).

19. David C. Thomasma, "An Analysis of Arguments For and Against Euthanasia and Assisted Suicide: Part One," *Cambridge Quarterly of Healthcare Ethics,* vol. 5, no. 1 (1996): 62–76.

20. Howard Brody, "Assisted Death—a Compassionate Response to a Medical Failure." *New England Journal of Medicine* 327 (1992): 1384–88.

21. Thomas Shannon and L. S. Cahill, *Religion and Artificial Reproduction* (New York: Crossroad, 1988).

22. David C. Thomasma and Erich H. Loewy, "A Dialogue on Species-Specific Rights: Human and Animals in Bioethics," *Cambridge Quarterly of Healthcare Ethics* vol. 6, no. 4 (1997): 435–44.

23. B. W. Rotzoll, "Woman, 80, First to Receive Fetal Eye Cells," *Chicago Sun-Times* (Feb. 1, 1997): 41.

24. Rotzoll, "Woman, 80, First to Receive Fetal Eye Cells." (Both quotes).

25. Leon Kass, "Neither For Love Nor Money: Why Doctors Must Not Kill," *Public Interest* 94 (1989): 25–46.

26. Kass, "Neither For Love Nor Money," 45.

27. Edmund Erde, "Person, Self, and Identity: A Metaphysical Deepening of Dilemmas in Medicine," *Theoretical Medicine and Bioethics,* in press.

28. Daniel Callahan, *Abortion, Law, Choice and Morality* (New York: Macmillan, 1970): 338.

29. Baruch Brody, *Abortion and the Sanctity of Human Life: A Philosophical View* (Cambridge, Mass. MIT Press, 1975): 40.

30. Brody, *Abortion and the Sanctity of Human Life,* 41.

31. See our analysis of such analogies with respect to taking the life of one conjoined twin to possibly save another: David C. Thomasma et al., "The Ethic of Caring For Conjoined Twins: The Lakeberg Twins," *Hastings Center Report,* vol. 26, no. 4 (1996): 4–12.

32. Most notable among these is H. Tristram Engelhardt, Jr., who has turned to religion for this foundation. See his *The Foundations of Bioethics,* 2nd ed. (New York: Oxford University Press, 1996).

33. Leo Tolstoy, "My Confession" in Emanuel Klemke, ed., *The Meaning of Life* (New York: Oxford University Press, 1981): 9–19. Quote: 15.

34. Tolstoy, "My Confession," 19.

35. David F. Swenson, "The Dignity of Human Life" in Klemke, *The Meaning of Life,* 20–30. Quote: 26.

36. Swenson, "The Dignity of Human Life," 27ff.

37. Engelhardt, *The Foundations of Bioethics.* Also Jonathan Moreno, *Deciding Together: Bioethics and Moral Consensus* (New York: Oxford University Press, 1995).

38. Engelhardt, *The Foundations of Bioethics.*

39. Peter Singer, *Rethinking Life and Death: The Collapse of Our Traditional Ethics* (New York: Oxford University Press, 1995).

40. Singer, *Rethinking Life and Death,* 75.

41. M. Therese Lysaught, " Suffering, Ethics, and the Body of Christ," *Christian Bioethics,* vol. 26, no. 2 (August 1996): 172–201. Quote: 193.

42. Bertrand B. Russell, "A Free Man's Workshop" in his *Why I Am Not A Christian* (New York: Simon & Schuster, 1957).

43. Albert Camus, *The Myth of Sisyphus and Other Essays,* trans. J. Obrien (New York: Alfred A. Knopf, Inc., 1955).

44. Julian Huxley, "I Believe" in Clifton Fadiman, ed., *I Believe* (New York: Simon & Schuster, 1939): 127–36.

45. Richard Taylor, *Good and Evil* (New York: Macmillan, 1970).

46. Judith Thomson, "A Defense of Abortion," *Philosophy and Public Affairs* 1 (1971): 47–66.

47. James Rachels, *The End of Life: Euthanasia and Morality* (New York: Oxford University Press, 1986).

48. Colman McCarthy, *All of One Peace: Essays on Nonviolence* (New Brunswick, N.J.: Rutgers University Press, 1994): 97.

Suffering and the Sufferer

The Meaning of Suffering: A Jewish Perspective

AVRAHAM STEINBERG, M.D.

DEFINITION OF TERMS

Human language has rich terminology to portray a wide variety of sufferings. Writers, poets, musicians, clergy, philosophers, social scientists, health-care workers, and others have depicted at length the essence of suffering in various forms and shapes.

In Hebrew there are several terms that describe various forms of physical and mental discomfort. *Suffering* (*yissurin*) originally denotes punishment,[1] or rebuke and moral teaching;[2] *soreness* (*ke'ev*) denotes subjective physical feeling that emanates from an illness or wound;[3] *burden* (*sevel*) metaphorically refers to carrying a heavy load of pain;[4,5] *affliction* (*eenuy*) refers to burden of fasting,[6] or burden of sexual assault;[7] and *pain* (*tzaar*) refers to the mental sensation of pain (talmudic expression).

SCIENTIFIC BACKGROUND

Pain and suffering are the most common complaints for which patients seek out physicians. Indeed, one of the central functions of medicine is to prevent, eliminate, or at least alleviate pain and suffering.

Biologically, pain sensation requires the presence of four conditions: pain receptors and pain sensation, nervous connections between the pain receptors and the nervous processing center, a nervous center to perceive the stimulus of pain, and the presence in the organism of a level of consciousness to be able to feel and to perceive pain.

Pain perception is a combination of physiological, psychological, mental, and behavioral interaction. It is dependent on an intact nervous system, and on subjective differences based on background, personality, culture, spirits, and circumstances. Pain can be aggravated by many subjective factors (i.e., fear, anxiety, depression, previous negative experiences, uncertainty, associated symptoms, nonsupportive environment).

Despite recent improvement in our understanding of pain mechanisms, however, pain perception is not yet adequately understood, and qualitative and quantitative pain measures are still unreliable.

The modern study of pain began about 150 years ago, but until the last few years, knowledge about the pathophysiology of pain was very limited. Therefore, effective pain-relieving measures were not used and there was inadequate awareness of the medical necessity to devote attention to patients' pain. In recent years there has been a significant improvement in pain treatment and management by pharmacological, surgical, and psycho-social measures. Currently, almost every pain can and should be treated and/or prevented. Treatment of physical pain alone is, however, not sufficient. In each instance the mental suffering should also be addressed.

CAUSES FOR SUFFERING

It is well established in Jewish writings that there is no human being without suffering. [8] However, one of the mysteries which Judaism has been grappling with since time immemorial is the issue of the purpose of suffering in the world. An even stronger enigma is the question "why the righteous suffer and the wicked have it good," [9,10,11] which is a bitter root for all disbelievers from all nations and peoples. [12]

Many explanations have been offered to elucidate these difficult questions. It seems reasonable that all explanations are partially correct. None, however, provides an entirely satisfactory answer.

A fundamental difference of opinion exists as to whether or not suffering occurs without sin. The talmudic expression of 'affliction of love for God' [13,14] is interpreted in different ways by those who feel that suffering exists without sin [15] and those who oppose such a possibility. [16]

One still needs to explain the essence and purpose of suffering, its timing, severity, and character. Many opinions and explanations have been offered.

SUFFERING AS PUNISHMENT AND ATONEMENT FOR SIN

Many biblical verses and talmudic statements indicate and emphasize this aspect. For example, "If you will not harken to the voice of the Lord thy God ... all these curses will come upon you"; [17] suffering comes because of bad deeds; [18] sufferings erase all persons' sins; [19] the moral-theological lesson of the story of Job is to stress that suffering comes to erase sins. [20] The thesis that suffering represents punishment and atonement for sin is also found in the writings of great Jewish scholars throughout the generations. This is particularly emphasized by Maimonides. [21]

SUFFERING BRINGS MAN CLOSER TO GOD AND TO PENITENCE

This thesis is enunciated in the Bible (and is also found in the Talmud). For example, "I found trouble and sorrow; then I called upon the name of the Lord"; [22] "Behold, happy is the man whom God rebukes." [23] The idea was further strengthened by later Jewish scholars, pointing out that the testing of Job was to bring him closer to God [24] and that suffering serves to remind a person to repent from his evil ways. [25]

SUFFERING AS A VEHICLE TO THE WORLD TO COME

This view is depicted by the rabbinic sages as follows: God brings sufferings on the righteous people in this world so that they inherit the world to come; [26] God inflicted sufferings on you in this world to cleanse you from your iniquities in the time to come; [27] Sufferings bring a person to the life in the world to come. [28] The view that suffering is a vehicle to bring one to the world to come is also found in the writings of great Jewish thinkers in later periods.

SUFFERING AS A "TRIAL"

A special chapter in the understanding of the purpose of suffering relates to the issue of trials. For example: "And God did tempt Abraham"; [29] "And He might prove thee to do thee good at thy latter end." [30] The purpose of such trials is highly debatable among Jewish scholars. Some opine that every trial cited in Scripture is to teach man what he ought to do or believe. [31] Other rabbis write that trials are to teach others the boundaries of the fear of God and to convert the good attributes of the righteous from potentiality to actuality to increase their reward. [32]

   After all is said, there is no good explanation for suffering and evil in the world, and there is no overall clarifying explanation which the human mind can understand. The comprehension of suffering is one of the great secrets of the Bible. Man cannot comprehend the ways of God and the reason for suffering. His rule over creatures is not the same as our rule over other beings. What is clear, however, is that suffering comes from God with divine righteousness. Suffering comes from God by Divine Providence for a purpose known to God, at a time, place, and degree determined by God, and with divine righteousness, as is stated in the Bible: "For all His ways are judgment, a God of truth and without iniquity, just and right is He." [33]

ATTITUDES TOWARD SUFFERING

According to most opinions of the talmudic sages and rabbinic scholars, one should not view suffering as having a lofty purpose by itself. Rather, suffering is an unwanted curse, even if it has a purpose. Therefore, the sages say that the life of a suffering person is no life. [34] It is, however, forbidden to allow suffering to pass without its leading to repentance. One should learn from suffering to improve one's deeds and repent for one's sins. [35] When pain and suffering occurs, even when it cannot be adequately controlled, the sages recommended the following attitudes: a person should always accustom himself to say that whatever the All-Merciful One does is for good; [36] if sufferings afflict a person, he should bear them, accept them, and he should not be resentful; [37] in spite of sufferings, one must love God, and strengthen his faith in God, as stated: "Though he slay me, yet I will trust in Him"; [38] "Shall we receive the good from God, and not receive the evil?" [39] In the final analysis, every sufferer should believe that it is because of his sins and iniquities, even though it might be the result of other causes.

Judaism's attitude toward suffering differs in many ways from other religions and philosophical/scientific approaches: Descartes [40] and subsequently the scientific community at large consider pain as a warning signal of imminent danger to the body. Therefore, the purpose of pain is to allow the diagnosis of the underlying problem and to correct it, in order to avoid the imminent injury or danger to a body organ or system. The problem with this view is that pain often does not indicate significant injury or danger. Furthermore, many life-threatening situations are not signaled by pain. Indeed, sometimes the pain itself is the major problem, not the injurious state. Judaism denies the notion that pain serves as a warning signal of imminent danger to the body. Hence, spiritual conclusions should also be derived from the experience of pain.

Most religions view pain to be the result of bad behavior and it serves as punishment for wrongdoing. In fact, the English word "pain" is derived from the Latin *paena* meaning punishment or payment. Moreover, Christianity views pain as the punishment for the original sin, and hence it is a welcomed experience, and it should not be prevented and should be gracefully accepted. Judaism accepts the idea that pain might be a punishment for sins. However, it negates the notion of original sin, and it certainly does not regard it as a virtue or sign of grace. Rather, pain and suffering is an unwanted curse, even if it has a purpose. Hence, it should be prevented and treated, including pangs of birth and death; self-imposition of afflictions, sufferings, and asceticism is not recommended and, in fact, forbidden.

Hinduism and Christian Science regard suffering as illusory and unreal, brought about by false beliefs and bad thinking and habits. Therefore, the goal of the sensation of pain is to change one's thoughts and beliefs and to see the world correctly. According to Judaism, suffering is real, not imaginative or illusory; hence, remedy should include physical/medical records.

CONCLUSIONS

- The comprehension of suffering is one of the great secrets of the Jewish faith. Man cannot comprehend the ways of God and the reason for suffering. His rule over creatures is not the same as our rule over other beings.
- After all is said, there is no explanation for suffering and evil in the world. What is clear, however, is that suffering comes from God by Divine Providence for a purpose known to God, at a time, place and degree determined by God, and with divine righteousness.
- On the one hand, pain and suffering should be treated medically and psychosocially in the most adequate way. On the other hand, it is forbidden to allow suffering to pass without its leading to repentance. One should learn from suffering to improve one's deeds and repent for one's sins.

NOTES

1. Deuteronomy 22:18.
2. Deuteronomy 8:5.
3. Genesis 34:25.
4. Genesis 49:15.
5. Isaiah 53:4.
6. Leviticus 23:29.
7. Deuteronomy 22:24.
8. Genesis Rabbah 92:1.
9. Jeremiah 12:1.
10. Ecclesiastes 7:15.
11. Berachot 7a.
12. Nachmanides, *Introduction to the Book of Job*.
13. Berachot 5a.

14. Shabbat 55a–b.
15. Rashi, *Berachot,* 5a; Bachaye, *Chovat Ha'Levavot, Shaar Ha'Bitachon,* 3.
16. Maimonides, *Guide of the Perplexed,* 3:17.
17. Deuteronomy 28:15.
18. Mishnah Kiddushin, 4:14.
19. Berachot 5a.
20. Maimonides, *Guide of the Perplexed,* 3:23.
21. Maimonides, *Guide of the Perplexed,* 3:17, 3:23.
22. Psalms 116:3–4.
23. Job 5:17.
24. Nachmanides, Job 38:1.
25. Shaare Teshiva, Shaar 2.
26. Kiddushin 40b.
27. Leviticus Rabbah 29:2.
28. Mechilta, Exodus 20:20.
29. Genesis 22:1.
30. Deuteronomy 8:16.
31. Maimonides, *Guide of the Perplexed,* 3:24.
32. Nachmanides, Torat Ha' Adam.
33. Deuteronomy 32:4.
34. Betzah 32b.
35. Ramban, Torat Ha' Adam; Rabbi J. B. Soloveitchik, *The Lonely Man of Faith* (New York: Doubleday, 1965).
36. Berachot 60b.
37. Genesis Rabbah 92:1.
38. Job 13:15.
39. Job 2:10.
40. Rene Descartes, "Meditation 6," in *Meditations* (New York: Liberal Arts Press, 1951).

The Meaning of Suffering?

REV. JAMES KEENAN, S.J., PH.D.

I begin my comments by noting that discussions on "the meaning of suffering" occur in two different contexts. The more familiar occurs in academic fora, which produce many philosophical and theological works about the "meaning of suffering." The less familiar occurs in those intimate settings in which someone suffering asks us for help in understanding her/his suffering; in that setting, we usually listen rather than talk.

In an academic impersonal context, there is less interest in the actual sufferer and more interest in the question of theodicy, that is, on how we can reconcile a merciful God with suffering. Most written works are not about sufferers but about God; they are addressed to a general audience philosophically or theologically interested in the topic rather than to those who are suffering. As a result these works tend to be theoretical and speculative, rather than practical. [1]

Daniel Simundson complements this insight about the context of such discussions in his important work, *Faith Under Fire*. There he notes that the Bible deals with suffering on two different levels: the intellectual level, where we "search for reasons *why* there is suffering in the world and *why* it comes to some and not to others," that is, the theodicy question, and the survival level, where we "provide support and comfort to the person who is experiencing suffering." [2] In the latter case, we rarely talk about the meaning of suffering; rather, we listen.

In light of these insights, I am not going to address the meaning of suffering as it generally is addressed, that is, academically. Rather, I ask how suffering should affect the delivery of health care. I ask what difference does suffering make to health care, or, what is the meaning of suffering for health care? Therefore, I do not look on my task as a philosophical investigation into theodicy, but as a response to one who is suffering. I want to examine what effect the testimony of sufferers has on health care providers. This is the "survival" discourse that Simundson talks about.

Toward this end, I begin by briefly commenting on how religion has responded to the fact of suffering. There I develop the importance of responding to suffering, predominantly by listening. Then I consider the role of the sufferer and the importance of his/her voice. Finally, I want to turn to the narrative of suffering as it should shape concretely the delivery of health care services. Thus, I want to use the topic "the meaning of suffering" to get us into a "listening mode" rather than a "speaking mode" with those who suffer.

RELIGIOUS RESPONSE TO SUFFERING

In his famous book, *Christ*, Edward Schillebeeckx describes how different secular and religious cultures address the question of suffering. Regarding religious societies, he remarks that while each religion has a different specific response in the face of suffering, they share "the fact that they give the last word to the *good*, and not to evil and suffering. None of them advocates a kind of dolorism; on the contrary, their deepest concern is to overcome suffering."[3] No religion then considers suffering as a good, per se; on the contrary, suffering is an enemy.

Of the many cultures he examines, I select three (one secular and two religious): those found in early Roman writings, the Hebrew Bible, and the Christian tradition. The Roman response to suffering is very different from religious ones. Considering suffering as a given, Romans made no attempt to find the cause of suffering. To be a human was itself a hard task, but any difficulties encountered were invitations to greatness, for the tragic became a way of conveying the hero. Though suffering itself was not a good, one's own response to suffering was what captured the Roman imagination.

In terms of Israel's response to suffering, Schillebeeckx remarks that whereas the Scriptures show that "Israel has no problems with suffering which men bring upon themselves through their own sinfulness . . . it protests and guards itself against unmerited suffering, quite independent of man's own folly." He adds, "Israel knew how to cope with suffering in religious terms; but sinfulness apart, it did not simply want to accept suffering as a *given*. The concept of fate is alien to Israel."[4] Nonetheless, Israel does suffer and without cause. Thus Schillebeeckx remarks that because of belief in God, "Israel did not hesitate to direct hard questions to God. 'Is God asleep?' asks Ps. 44.23, 26." Reviewing a few additional passages from the Hebrew Bible, Schillebeeckx concludes, "faith in God, the author of good and opponent of all evil, i.e., faith that good has the last word, becomes the fundamental attitude of Israel, though at the same time it cherishes a protest because all this has taken so long." [5]

Finally, Christians see God and suffering as "diametrically opposed; where God appears, evil and suffering have to yield. So there is no place for suffering. . . ." Moreover, Schillebeeckx remarks that Jesus "breaks with the idea that suffering necessarily has something to do with sinfulness." Looking at the Johannine description of the man born blind (John 9:2f) and the Lucan account of the murdered Galileans (Luke 13:1–5) we see "that it is possible to draw conclusions from sin to suffering, but not from suffering to sin." Schillebeeckx discusses at length the Christian notion of redemptive suffering, though he notes its misuse. Instead he argues that the redemptive and ultimately truly liberating significance of suffering lies in the suffering which a person has to assume in one's responsible concern to overcome suffering. [6]

That particular election aside, Schilleebeckx notes what all religions have in common. "All religions have made a zealous quest for the causes of suffering precisely in order to remove these causes by following a particular course of action." [7] That is, the answer to the question of "why do I suffer" is raised not to find meaning, but to find the cause so as to remove it. In other words, the religious response to suffering is to find out a way of eliminating suffering. On the other hand, he adds that aside from contemporary Marxists, secularized Europeans, like the earlier Romans, neither seek the cause of suffering nor protest against it. [8] Thus peculiar to the investigation of suffering by religious believers is the pursuit of suffering for the purpose of eliminating it.

Schillebeeckx provides strong testimony regarding Christian faith and suffering that in some circles is often misunderstood. Though he acknowledges that some suffering may actually help some individuals to become more sensitive and compassionate and, in some instances, actually transform a person, still he says decisively, "there is an excess of suffering and evil in our history. There is a barbarous excess, for all the explanations and interpretations. There is too much *unmerited* and *senseless* suffering for us to be able to give an ethical, hermeneutical and ontological analysis of our disaster." He surmises, "human reason cannot in fact cope with concentrated historical suffering and evil." [9] But neither can Scriptures explain away suffering. He writes:

> The Christian message does not give an *explanation* of evil or our history of suffering. That must be made clear from the start. Even for Christians, suffering remains impenetrable and incomprehensible, and provokes rebellion. Nor will the Christian blasphemously claim that God himself

required the death of Jesus as compensation for what *we* make of our history. [10]

Schillebeeckx is helpful here. He describes convincingly a variety of religious responses to suffering that are each truly representative of the religion he describes. He also corrects those false impressions of Christianity, which too often Christians promote, that seem to make suffering an expression of a loving God's will. But he leaves us short on two points. First, secular society does look for the cause of suffering. The entire conflict between religion and medicine is precisely based on the latter resisting the former's norms for eliminating suffering. Medicine and religion have conflicted in part because both are interested in discovering the cause and the cure for suffering. [11] Second, he makes too much of "unmerited" suffering. Certainly, Schillebeeckx acknowledges that Job, like Luke and John, demonstrates that we cannot induce sin from suffering. Nonetheless, the connection between the two remains a problem for Schillebeeckx. [12] How are we to determine the difference between "merited" and "unmerited" suffering? How can we know that someone's suffering is really "unmerited"? Does the AIDS victim have to be a child or a hemophiliac? Does the cancer victim really have to have been taking every precaution against carcinogens? Does the tortured political activist really have to be politically prudent? Does the date rape victim really have to be insisting on "No" the entire evening?

The distinction between merited and unmerited suffering strikes me as still engaging the albeit modified stance of Eliphaz, Bildad, and Zophar who contended with Job about his "merited suffering." [13] My point is, if we believers only stand in protest against unmerited suffering, how are we to know what is and what isn't merited? And, if we insist on the distinction, it seems to me that a deep residue of moralism is apparent wherever listeners are encouraged to sift out the "merited" from "unmerited" sufferers.

In making these points, let me add two further comments. First, I am not denying that some suffering is tragically unmerited; for believers that is the great question for God and about theodicy. [14] That the suffering is unmerited is something that the sufferer per se knows. Generally speaking, the listener or onlooker is unable to mediate the claims of suffering as merited or unmerited. Moreover, I fail to see what difference merit makes, if we ask about the meaning of suffering for health care. The health care provider does not determine whose suffering merits attention and whose does not. The stance of the health care provider before the face of the suffering person is not to be a discerning moralizer but rather to be an attentive listener and respondent. This does not mean, however, that a person's previous or predictable future conduct does not enter into triage considerations. For instance, we may make some decisions about a liver transplant differently for one who is a chronic alcoholic from one who is not. But our only reason for that decision is not based on merit, but on forecast, not based on moral judgment, but pragmatic judgment. We simply estimate how successful a liver transplant will be in one patient as opposed to another.

These reservations aside, we learn from Schillebeeckx that religion prompts us to respond to the sufferer by trying to find the cause of her or his suffering. Toward this end, the first stance of the respondent is, as Schillebeeckx urges, to listen. [15] Likewise, when Simundson examines the survival level response to suffering, he argues that the primary biblical recommendation is to allow the sufferer to lament. [16] In this case he finds in particular that the Hebrew Bible is especially instructive.

LISTENING

Before turning again to the Scriptures, I think we need to recognize the critical importance of listening to the sufferer in order to assist the health care provider in understanding what exactly is affecting the sufferer. Listening is all the more important when the sufferer is not immediately forthcoming about the sufferer's own well-being. This seems to be, in fact, a commonplace. In a source that I am unable to remember or locate, I read that in many patient interviews, patients do not name their major ailment until they first mention one or two lesser ones. That is, initially, the first two items reported by some patients are not the reasons for the patient's visit, whereas the third item is. Thus, on occasion, the inattentive or rushed physician sends home a patient who never utters the real reason for his/her concern. Let me make a curious aside. In my training for hearing confessions, I was similarly informed that it is not until the third confessed sin that the penitent gets down to serious sins. Not uncommonly we hear things like, "I swore, I missed mass, I committed adultery, I was testy at work."

Still, there is something more integral for responding to suffering than simply hearing the correct ailment. That is, the act of listening encourages the sufferer to speak. Encouraging the sufferer to speak is a very biblical stance. In a rather brilliant article, J. David Pleins addresses the issue of the "Divine Silence" in Job. Pleins argues that unlike those so-called friends of Job who do not allow him to speak and who try to redirect the purpose of his discourse, God allows Job to speak. Not God's absence but "God's silence dominates the discussions of Job with his friends." [17] The same listening stance is also apparent in those who stood helpless at the cross of Jesus and who heard his words, even his cry to God, "My God, my God, why have you forsaken me?" They, like God, listen to the cry of the sufferer. Of course, in the face of God's silence we, like the psalmist, might ask God, "Are you asleep?" But God's silence both in Job and at the crucifixion seems to convey a God who is both attentive and listening.

This listening stands as an alternative to the Christian urge to interpret in the face of suffering. For some Christians differentiate suffering from pain precisely in that, as Joseph Selling argues, "pain demands a response, while suffering demands an interpretation." [18] Yet it has been the Christian urge to translate or interpret another's suffering that has led in this decade to some really terrible remarks. I think here specifically of unfortunate moments when certain Catholic leaders, known for wanting to better Christian-Jewish relations, let their own theology of suffering interpret the Jewish suffering in the Holocaust. [19] Worse still is the insistence of Christians to speak about another's suffering, especially when they were the cause of that suffering. Marcel Sarot brings this point out poignantly in his "Auschwitz, Morality and the Suffering of God." [20] There Sarot calls upon his fellow Christian theologians to declare a moratorium on raising up Auschwitz as providing testimony necessary to understand faith and suffering. In particular he cites numerous instances of Christians translating or interpreting the meaning of Jewish questions and answers in the aftermath of Auschwitz. He especially addresses the Christian insistence to answer the Jewish sufferer who asks, "Where is God in all this?" Sarot contends that the primary question that Christians should raise in the face of Auschwitz is not "What concept of God gives most comfort to those who suffer?" Rather, Auschwitz should prompt Christians to ask "How can we prevent Christianity from ever again providing fertile soil for antisemitism and kindred movements?" [21]

The Christian insistence on interpreting in the face of suffering must be challenged by the Jewish insistence on listening. Like Simundson and Sarot, Paul Nelson argues that "Christians would do better to face up to the pointlessness of this attitude taking a lesson from the Hebrew scriptures. The psalms of lament . . . make no attempt to explain or palliate. Instead they give voice to human anguish, rage and despair on the apparent assumption that the God of Israel is strong enough to take it." [22]

Apart from the religious prescription to encourage lament, the need for the sufferer to express her/his suffering is manifold. As Eric Cassell, author of *The Nature of Suffering* [23] has made clear, "suffering is necessarily private because it is ultimately individual." [24] Like others, Cassell distinguishes pain from suffering inasmuch as the former can exist without the latter and conversely. He describes suffering as "the distress brought about by the actual or perceived impending threat to the integrity or continued existence of the whole person." [25] Suffering begins not so much when we become aware of the fact that we cannot do something, but rather when we become aware of what our future holds. Suffering arises with "the loss of the ability to pursue purpose." [26] Thus, in the face of such vulnerability, we face the loss of a self who organizes purposeful action. The loss of our ability to pursue our purposes is the basis of our suffering. But beneath that ground is what Sebastian MacDonald calls, "a drive to survive." [27] Thus, to appreciate what exactly is the suffering of a particular person, we must understand not only the facts of loss, but two other more individual and more subjective considerations. First, we must understand how that loss fits into the world of values that the sufferer has purposefully pursued, that is, what she/he specifically fears is threatened. Second, we must understand the world of relations in which the sufferer continues to endure the threats to self, that is, the way the sufferer pursues her/his survival. We can only understand these subjective considerations if we allow the sufferer to pursue her/his survival. Thus, we can only respond to suffering by listening.

VOICE

The call for the respondent to listen to one who is suffering is not necessarily an easy one, for it presupposes that the sufferer can or will speak. Meredith McGuire reminds us, for instance, that pain unites the body and mind, but despite this connection, suffering results precisely because the body in pain is often unable to express itself. [28] Paul Brand captures this phenomenon by considering chronic pain and its inability to free the sufferer to speak. Pain inhibits the sufferer from doing the only thing that the sufferer wants to do: communicate her pain. [29] Brand offers some resolution by highlighting the empathetic quality of pain and by demonstrating that the witness to one in pain can sometimes communicate and articulate the depth of the suffering. That is, Brand still tries to have the interlocutor "listen" to another who is suffering even when the sufferer cannot speak. Likewise, Cassell invites medical practitioners to develop an aesthetic sense by which they can try to apprise the suffering of another who cannot speak but who communicates her suffering through a variety of movements. [30] This aesthetic sense can only be developed when the listener is attentive to the nature of suffering in her/his own life. Thus, in *At the Will of the Body*, Arthur Frank engages us to become aware of the narrative of pain within our own bodies and so invites us to give voice to our own pain, hopefully assisting us to learn to listen to another's own narrative of suffering. [31] Revisiting the terrain of one's own past suffering establishes the groundwork for becoming a compassionate and perceptive listener. [32]

That the body becomes the expresser of suffering is very important. Rejecting any soul and body dualism, [33] we should recognize that where there is no voice to express the suffering that, as Eli Yasif claims, "the body never lies." [34] Nonetheless, the body, in all its pain and suffering, seeks to express itself through the voice. Thus, even when the sufferer cannot voice in any *articulate* way her/his suffering, still the voice may be able to *utter* its suffering. Barbara Bozak thus turns to the Psalms of Lament as a means by which one in pain can begin to utter the depth of her/his suffering. [35] With these psalms, the sufferer, unable to express or name the particularity of her/his suffering, is still able to acknowledge to some extent its depth. Likewise, reciting the Psalms for one unable to speak enables at least the sufferer's surrogate voice to speak.

Nowhere has the relationship between the voice and suffering been better captured than in *The Body in Pain: The Making and Unmaking of the World,* where Elaine Scarry examines torture. She cogently argues that torturers derive their power from the voices of the tortured. She explains that the object of torture is not to exact a confession nor to learn information, but rather to force the tortured person to accuse her/his very self; the tortured voice betrays the body when, so broken with pain, the body is unable to keep the voice from submitting to the fictive power of the torturer. The aim of torture, then, is dualism: to tear the voice from its body: "The goal of the torturer is to make the one, the body, emphatically and crushingly *present* by destroying it, and to make the other, the voice, *absent* by destroying it." The tortured body is left voiceless, once it acknowledges the torturer's power. [36] Separating the voice from the body is the object of those who deliberately cause suffering. Those who want to make another suffer recognize that the unitive element for a person of purpose is the voice. They torture to the point that their victim's voice becomes the accuser.

Scarry notes that the tortured person's most difficult wound to heal is the voice. For this reason Amnesty International assists the tortured, unable out of shame to tell their narratives, to read and understand their records so that they may one day articulate the truth of the atrocities. Scarry's work convincingly demonstrates the centrality of the human voice in attaining healing integration. Together with the other writers, she highlights that silencing and other forms of exclusion are physically and personally destructive acts.

DIRECTIVES FOR HEALTH CARE

This study into the meaning of suffering has led us to see, hopefully, several important insights that ought to directly affect health care.

First, inasmuch as suffering is a private act, we can only understand a person's suffering if we allow the sufferer to communicate.

Second, as opposed to the more prevalent tendency of Christians to interpret or translate suffering, Jewish writers, both with and without the Hebrew Scriptures, insist upon the importance of listening to the sufferer.

Third, the act of listening itself is troublesome particularly because the terrors and the trauma associated with the threat and the loss experienced in suffering often inhibit the sufferer from intelligibly articulating the cause and/ or depth of suffering. Moreover, the voice itself, not merely the sufferer's intelligence, is also, especially in times of pain, muted. Thus when the voice is unable to express itself, the sufferer loses finally the most integral way by which a sufferer can communicate and remain in contact with the community that supports her/him. Progressively, studies show us not only the therapeutic function that the voice has in the life of the sufferer, but conversely the compounded suffering that occurs when the voice is ignored, lost, or silenced. For like torture itself, the act of silencing a sufferer, or worse, of making a suffering person speak against herself/himself is a violent action.

Though there have been ample writings on the meaning of suffering, many of them violate the sufferer yet again, to the extent that they ignore, replace, or translate the sufferer's own voice without heeding exactly what the narrator has communicated. I think, for instance, of the Christian insistence on translating the suffering of the Jews in the Holocaust. Likewise, I think of the suffering of homosexuals in the Holocaust who have rarely been given a hearing. But while religious communities and religious leaders as well as others have violated the suffering of many by their broad reworking of the sufferers' narratives, that same violence occurs again and again in the habitual acts in the medical profession wherein physicians and nurses ignore, silence, translate, or belittle the voices of their patients. [37]

I cannot in the time allotted make more than brief comments as to what the practice of giving patients their voice and respecting their narratives concretely means. I can refer you to the dated but helpful and bibliographically rich essay by Karen Lebacqz titled, "The Virtuous Patient." [38] I also recommend Dr. Pellegrino's *The Virtues in Medical Practice.* [39] To their important insights, I add that the meaning of suffering for health care is that it requires those responding to the patient to first and foremost encourage her/him to speak, to voice both the cause and narrative of her/his suffering. This requires, in turn, a compassionate attentiveness and a willing listening stance on the part of the provider. This also requires the narrative of a sufferer's testimony to be treated respectfully. This I cannot underline enough.

Finally, taking the stance of listener to the suffering patient, health care providers must rethink the way that they make decisions regarding the delivery of health care. To make this point, I refer to an important shift that can be found in the recently revised "Ethical and Religious Directives for Catholic Health Care Services." [40] Despite the fact that my friend and colleague Kevin Wildes has written in the *Kennedy Institute of Ethics Journal* that the "Directives offer little that is new," [41] these Directives rejected the previously mandated best-interests model for authorizing health care decisions in favor of the patient-wishes model. As opposed to the best-interests model that leaves to physicians and others, including surrogates, the decision to determine proper care for a patient according to the proverbial "medical indications," the patient-wishes model requires that wherever ethical options in health care exist, the patient is the final arbiter. Moreover, in the event that the patient loses competency, then the surrogate must be "faithful to the patient's intention" and in the event there are no advanced directives, then the staff must consult the person who is in the position "to know best the patient's wishes." The Directives go so far as to argue that the determination of extraordinary means is a patient's judgment. During many rewrites, the Vatican asked the American drafting committee whether they did not want to return what the Vatican considered was the morally safer "best-interests" model. The bishops resisted, arguing that the five Directives (25, 26, 27, 28, and 32) affected by the shift were framed by the repeated insistence (Directives 5–9, 24, 28) that no Catholic health care facility would honor a request specifically contrary to the Directives, e.g., abortion or assisted suicide. Still, for the first time, bishops were throwing aside a legacy of paternalism in health care and insisting that patients have not only a voice, but the final say in their own health care.

But if this essay has been on listening to the sufferer, it may be most fitting to close with two stories from a patient and from her mother. Connie is a lawyer friend of mine and a devoted mother of three, whose middle daughter is an eleven-year-old fighting leukemia. She told me the story of a little eight-year-old in the bed next to her daughter who was also suffering from leukemia. A nurse came in to give the girl an injection and the girl cried, "I'm afraid." "No, you're not afraid, you are a big girl," said the nurse in contradiction, giving the girl her injection. After the nurse left, my friend Connie went over to the girl's mother and said, "Excuse me, but I would never let a nurse or doctor contradict my child. Things are bad enough without her having to conform her suffering to the nurse's efficiency."

The second one is like the first. Connie's daughter, Maureen, suffering from punctured lungs, has been living for several weeks with tubes in her chest. An older women in her room had a similar catheter. The older woman said to Maureen, "Honey, when they put that thing in your chest, did they say that you would experience 'discomfort'?" "Yes," she responded. "You know, discomfort is sitting in a wooden chair for twenty minutes or wearing tight shoes. That thing hanging out of your chest isn't discomfort; it's living hell." Little Maureen, facing leukemia, found in that woman someone who knew her suffering. But those who translated her suffering as "discomfort" were unable to listen, let alone understand the little girl's living hell.

In a word, the humanization of medicine will only occur when we allow the narratives of suffering together with the language of the sufferer to shape the care we deliver.

NOTES

1. See such diverse writings as Thomas Aquinas, *The Literal Exposition on Job* (Atlanta: Scholar's Press, 1989): 223–31; Mother Angelica, "Why Do We Suffer?" *Mother Angelica's Answers, Not Promises* (New York: Harper and Row, 1989): 60–89.

2. Daniel Simundson, *Faith under Fire* (Minneapolis: Augsburg Publishing House, 1980): 144.

3. Edward Schillebeeckx, *Christ* (New York: Seabury Press, 1980): 675.

4. Schillebeeckx, *Christ*, 677.

5. Schillebeeckx, *Christ*, 678.

6. Schillebeeckx, *Christ*, 694–700. Here there is something distinctive about Christian notions of suffering that though not directly applicable to the issue of suffering and medical care is still noteworthy. Here is love electing suffering and the primary model for this love is God. On this point, William Placher rather eloquently addresses the vulnerability of God and notes with Dietrich Bonhoeffer that, "God suffers because God is vulnerable, and God is vulnerable because God loves—and it is love, not suffering or even vulnerability, that is finally the point. . . . The freedom of love is good, and that freedom risks suffering and, in a sinful world full of violence and injustice, will always encounter it sooner or later. Love does not regret the price it pays for making itself vulnerable, but to speak of paying a price is itself to acknowledge that the suffering is itself an evil. Vulnerability, on the other hand, is a perfection of loving freedom." William Placher, *Narratives of a Vulnerable God* (Louisville: Westminster, 1994): 18–19. Much less satisfying is Stanley Hauerwas, "Reflections on Suffering, Death and Medicine," *Suffering Presence* (Notre Dame: University of Notre Dame Press, 1986): 23–38.

7. Schillebeeckx, *Christ*, 715.

8. Schillebeeckx, *Christ,* 718.

9. Schillebeeckx, *Christ,* 724–25.

10. Schillebeeckx, *Christ,* 728.

11. See Darrel Amundsen and Gary Ferngren's essays, "Virtue and Health/ Medicine in Pre-Christian Antiquity," "Virtue and Medicine from Early Christianity through the Sixteenth Century," Earl E. Shelp, ed., *Virtue and Medicine* (Dordrecht; Boston: D. Reidel, 1985): 3–22, 23–62.

12. There is, of course, the problem of what a sin really is. I have addressed this issue looking, for instance, at the casualness with which the Christian tradition has called wrong behavior "sinful." Is the adolescent who masturbates a sinner? Is an alcoholic a sinner? Is the manically depressed? Is wrong behavior really as sinful as it is usually described? And if so, is every instance of wrong behavior one that results in merited suffering? See my "The Problem with Thomas Aquinas's Concept of Sin," *Heythrop Journal* 35 (1994): 401–20.

13. Mother Angelica, "Why Do We Suffer?", 60–89.

14. See Herman-Emiel Mertens, "The Loving God and the Suffering Human," *Louvain Studies* 16 (1991): 170–77.

15. Schillebeeckx, *Christ,* 722.

16. See Simundson, *Faith under Fire,* 43–61, 148–50.

17. J. David Pleins, "'Why Do You Hide Your Face?' Divine Silence and Speech in the Book of Job," *Interpretation* 48 (July 1994): 230.

18. Joseph Selling, "A Credible Response to the Meaning of Suffering," Jan Lambrecht and Raymond Collins eds., *God and Human Suffering* (Louvain: Peeters, 1990): 181; quoted in Mertens, 175.

19. See one rabbi's response to the pope, Robert Hirschfield, "Rabbi Marshall Meyer: A Prophet's Agenda," *The Christian Century* 106 (26 April 1989): 438–39.

20. Marcel Sarot, "Auschwitz, Morality and the Suffering of God," *Modern Theology* 7 (1991): 135–52.

21. Sarot, "Auschwitz, Morality and the Suffering of God," 139.

22. Paul Nelson, "The Problem of Suffering," *The Christian Century* 108 (May 1, 1991): 491.

23. Eric Cassell, *The Nature of Suffering* (New York: Oxford University Press, 1991).

24. Cassell, "Recognizing Suffering," *Hastings Center Report* 21 (1991): 31.

25. Cassell, "Recognizing Suffering," 24.

26. Cassell, "Recognizing Suffering," 25.

27. Sebastian MacDonald, *Moral Theology and Suffering* (New York: Peter Lang, 1995): 9–18.

28. See Meredith McGuire, "Religion and the Body," *The Journal for the Scientific Study of Religion* 29 (1990): 283–96, 287–89.

29. Paul Brand, *In His Image* (Grand Rapids: Zondervan, 1987): 226–91.

30. Cassell, "Recognizing Suffering," 24–31.

31. Arthur Frank, *At the Will of the Body* (New York: Houghton Miflin, 1992).

32. MacDonald, *Moral Theology and Suffering,* 19–46.

33. See my "Christian Perspectives on the Human Body," *Theological Studies* 55 (1994): 330–46; "Dualism in Medicine, Christian Theology and the Aging," *Journal of Religion and Health,* forthcoming.

34. Eli Yasif, "The Body Never Lies: The Body in Medieval Jewish Folk Narratives," Howard Eilberg-Schwartz, *People of the Body: Jews and Judaism from an Embodied Perspective* (Albany: State University of New York Press, 1992): 203–22.

35. Barbara Bozak, "Suffering and the Psalms of Lament," *Eglise et Theologie* 23 (1992): 325–38.

36. Elaine Scarry, *The Body in Pain: The Making and Unmaking of the World* (New York: Oxford University Press, 1985): 27–59.

37. See the helpful essays, Matthew Budd and Michael Zimmerman, "The Potentiating Clinician: Combining Scientific and Linguistic Competence," *Advances* 3 (1986): 40–55; Larry Churchill and Sandra Churchill, "Storytelling in Medical Arenas: The Art of Self-Determination," ed., Kathryn Rabuzzi, *Literature and Medicine* 1 (1982): 73–9; Kathryn Montgomery Hunter, "Paradigms and the Patient-Doctor Encounter," *Advances* 10 (1994): 51–54; ibid., "Remaking the Case," *Literature and Medicine* 11, (1992): 163–79; Anton Kuzel, "Naturalistic Inquiry: An Appropriate Model for Family Medicine," *Family Medicine* 18 (1986): 369–74.

38. Karen Lebacqz, "The Virtuous Patient" in *Virtue and Medicine*, ed. Earl E. Shelp (Dordrecht; Boston: D. Reidel, 1985): 275–86.

39. Edmund Pellegrino and David Thomasma, *The Virtues in Medical Practice* (New York: Oxford University Press, 1993).

40. U.S. Bishops, "Ethical and Religious Directives for Catholic Health Care Services," *Origins* 24 (1994): 449–61.

41. Kevin Wildes, "A Memo from the Central Office: The Ethical and Religious Directives for Catholic Health Care Services," *Kennedy Institute of Ethics Journal* 5 (1995): 133–40.

SECTION FOUR

Healing and the Healer

The Imperative to Heal in Traditional Judaism

FRED ROSNER, M.D., F.A.C.P.

INTRODUCTION

In the Jewish tradition, a physician is given specific divine license to practice medicine. Not only is the physician permitted and even obligated to minister to the sick, but the patient is obligated to care for his health and life. Another cardinal principle in Judaism is that human life is of infinite value. The preservation of human life takes precedence over all but three biblical commandments: the prohibitions against idolatry, murder, and forbidden sexual relations such as incest and adultery. In order to preserve a human life, the Sabbath and even the Day of Atonement may be desecrated, and all other rules and laws (save the above three) are suspended for the overriding consideration of saving a human life.

Judaism never condones the deliberate destruction of human life except in judicial execution for certain criminal acts, in self-defense, or in time of war. One may also not sacrifice one life to save another life or even many other lives. Many of the principles of Jewish medical ethics are based on this concept of the infinite value of human life. He who saves one life, asserts the Talmud,[1] is as if he saved a whole world. For every person even a few moments of life are worthwhile.

How far does the physician's obligation to heal extend? Is the physician obligated to endanger his own life to treat patients with contagious and/or communicable diseases? How much risk to his own health and life is the physician allowed or obligated to undertake in the care of his patients? Does the general obligation to visit the sick also include visits to patients with contagious or infectious diseases?

THE PHYSICIAN'S IMPERATIVE TO HEAL

The ethical and legal question of whether or not a person is allowed or obligated under Jewish law to become a physician and heal the sick is based on the biblical statement in which God asserts: "I am the Lord that heals you" [2] which, literally translated from the Hebrew, means I am the Lord, your physician. If God states that he is the healer of the sick, how can we, as human physicians, play God, so to speak? The answer is found later in the Bible where the duplicate mention of healing in the phrase "and heal he shall heal" [3] is interpreted by the sages of the Talmud [4] to mean that authorization was granted by God to a physician to heal. The Bible implies that it is as if there are two physicians: one is Almighty God, the true healer of the sick, and the other is the human physician who serves as an instrument of God or an extension of God in the ministrations to the sick.

Many biblical commentators echo this talmudic teaching. By the insistence or emphasis expressed in the double wording, "heal he shall heal," the Bible opposes the erroneous idea that having recourse to medicine shows lack of trust and faith in divine assistance. The Bible takes it for granted that medical therapy is used and actually requires it. Other biblical and rabbinic sources which address the physician's obligation to heal are discussed at length elsewhere. [5,6]

THE PATIENT'S OBLIGATION TO SEEK HEALING

A physician is divinely licensed and biblically obligated to heal the sick because of the Jewish concept of the supreme value of human life. Is a patient, however, authorized or perhaps mandated to seek healing from a physician? Is a patient who asks a physician to heal him denying Divine Providence? Is illness an affliction from God that serves as punishment for wrongdoing?

The strongest evidence in Jewish sources that a patient is permitted to seek healing from a physician is found in Maimonides' Code of Jewish Law, known as *Mishneh Torah,* [7] as follows:

A person should set his heart that his body be healthy and strong in order that his soul be upright to know the Lord. For it is impossible for man to understand and comprehend the wisdoms [of the world] if he is hungry and ailing or if one of his limbs is aching.

Numerous talmudic citations indicate that patients are allowed and even required to seek medical attention. In Jewish tradition, the patient is obligated to care for his health and life. He is charged with preserving his health. He must eat and drink and sustain himself and must seek healing when he is ill in order to be able to serve the Lord in a state of good health. One might arrive at the same conclusion if one were to interpret literally the biblical admonition, "Take therefore good heed unto yourselves." [8]

THE PHYSICIAN'S OBLIGATION TO HEAL PATIENTS WITH CONTAGIOUS DISEASES

How far does the physician's divine mandate to heal the sick extend? Is a physician obligated to treat a patient with a contagious disease if there is a risk that he may contract the illness from the patient? Is a physician obligated to endanger his own health or life to restore the health or save the life of the patient?

Jewish law requires that if one sees one's neighbor drowning or being mauled by beasts or attacked by robbers, he is bound to save him. [9] This rule is codified by Maimonides [10] and Karo. [11] Elsewhere, Karo rules [12] that if one observes a ship sinking with people on board, or a river overflowing its banks, thereby endangering lives, or a pursued person whose life is in danger, one is obligated to desecrate the Sabbath to save the victims. The commentaries of Rabbi Israel Meir Kagan (1838–1933) [13] and Rabbi Abraham Zvi Hirsch Eisenstadt (1813–1868) [14] add that if there is danger involved to the rescuer, the latter is *not* obligated to endanger his life because his life takes precedence over that of his fellow man. If there is only a small risk to the rescuer, he should carefully evaluate the potential danger to himself and act accordingly.

How should a physician proceed if the patient is suffering from a contagious disease? Is the physician allowed to refuse to treat the patient because of the risk or because of his fear of contracting the disease? What if the risk is very small? What is the definition of small risk? If there is a significant risk to the physician contracting the disease from his patient, Jewish law would certainly agree that the physician would not be obligated to care for that patient. If he wished to care for the patient despite the risk, his act is considered to be a pious act by some writers, and folly by others. If the risk is very remote, however, the physician must care for the patient.

The question as to whether or not a person is obligated or allowed to subject himself to risk in order to save another's life is related to the well-known difference of opinion between the Babylonian and Jerusalem Talmuds. The Jerusalem Talmud [15] posits that a person is obligated to potentially endanger his life if the risk is small to save the life of a fellow human being from certain danger. On the other hand, the Babylonian Talmud [16] voices the opinion that a person is not obligated but is allowed to endanger his life if the risk is small, to save the life of another.

The prevailing opinion among the various rabbinic sources is the one cited by Rabbi David Ibn Zimra (1479–1573). [17] If there is great danger to the rescuer, he is not allowed to attempt to save his fellow man; if he nevertheless does so, he is called a pious fool. If the danger to the rescuer is small and the danger to his fellow man very great, the rescuer is allowed but not obligated to attempt the rescue, and if he does so his act is called an act of loving kindness. If there is no risk at all to the rescuer or if the risk is very small or remote, he is obligated to try to save his fellow man. If he refuses to do so, he is guilty of transgressing the commandment, "Thou shalt not stand idly by the blood of thy fellow man." [18] This approach is also adopted by recent rabbinic deciders, including Rabbi Moshe Feinstein [19] and Rabbi Eliezar Yehuda Waldenberg. [20] Since the risk to physicians and other health care personnel in caring for patients with contagious diseases such as tuberculosis, or communicable diseases such as acquired immunodeficiency syndrome (AIDS) is very small if one takes the necessary precautions, a physician is obligated under Jewish law to care for such patients.

Medical history and tradition are replete with examples of physicians whose devotion to their patients transcended their concern for any possible personal danger of contracting their patients' diseases. Physicians caring for patients with plague, cholera, typhoid, and polio occasionally became victims themselves. Throughout the ages, the physician's obligations not only to his patients but to society, other health professionals, and to himself have not always been accepted as axiomatic. The profound reluctance of some physicians to care for patients with AIDS prompted Zuger and Miles to review medical responses to other historic plagues. [21] Many physicians, including Galen from Rome in the second century and Sydenham from London in the seventeenth century fled from patients with contagious epidemic diseases. Many of their colleagues, at considerable personal risk, remained behind to care for plague victims.

In Jewish sources, the nearly universal recommendation for those threatened by plague is flight: "He that remains in the city shall die ... by the pestilence, but he that goes out ... he shall live." [22] The Talmud states that if one finds one's self in a pestilence-ridden town, "gather your feet," [23] which means to flee, or to withdraw to a safe place. During an epidemic of plague, Raba used to close his window shutters [24] because, as Jeremiah [25] lamented: "Death is come up unto our windows."

Jakobovits points out that it was customary in medieval Jewish communities not to assign visitation of plague-stricken patients to anyone except specially appointed persons who were well paid for their perilous work. [26] He also cites the seventeenth-century records of the Portuguese Congregation in

Hamburg, which indicate that even the communal physicians and nurses were exempt from the obligation to attend to infectious patients and that the required services were rendered by volunteers entitled to special remuneration.

The risk of contracting AIDS by examining the patient is extremely small. Hence, Judaism requires physicians and others to care for such patients. Precautions, wherever possible, must be taken by all health care personnel to minimize the chances of sticking or cutting themselves or others with a scalpel or needle that has been used to draw blood from an AIDS patient.

The American Medical Association Council on Ethical and Judicial Affairs stresses doctors' duty to AIDS patients by stating that:

- A physician may not ethically refuse to treat a patient whose condition is within the physician's current realm of competence solely because the patient is seropositive. Persons who are seropositive should not be subjected to discrimination based on fear or prejudice.
- Physicians are dedicated to providing competent medical service with compassion and respect for human dignity.
- Physicians who are unable to provide the services required by AIDS patients should make referrals to those physicians or facilities equipped to provide such services.

The American College of Physicians and the Infectious Diseases Society of America believe that physicians, other health care professionals, and hospitals are obligated to provide competent and humane care to all patients, including patients with AIDS and AIDS-related conditions as well as HIV-infected patients with unrelated problems. The denial of appropriate care to patients for any reason is unethical. [27] The Association of American Medical Colleges has also adopted a statement concerning the professional responsibility in treating AIDS patients. [28]

The law cannot force people and/or physicians to be courageous or virtuous. [29] Moreover, society cannot expect physicians and health care providers to be saints and/or martyrs. The professional obligation of a physician based on the devotion to the moral ideal of healing the sick has some constraints. Physicians are obviously not obligated to treat a patient whose disease and therapy are beyond their competence. Other limiting factors include excessive risk, minimal or questionable benefits, existing obligations to other patients, and competing obligations to family and self. [30]

The consensus of opinion seems to be that a person assumes a unique responsibility when he enters a healing profession. "Having accepted the mantle of physician, we are no longer absolutely free to choose which patients we will and will not treat." [31] In this respect, medicine differs from business and most other careers and, therefore, imposes an obligation of effacement of self-interest on the physician. These differences of "the nature of illness, the non-proprietary character of medical knowledge, and the oath of fidelity to the patient's interests generate strong moral obligations." [32]

CONCLUSION

According to the precepts of Judaism, every human life is infinitely valuable. Therefore, physicians and other health care providers are obligated to endeavor to heal the sick and prolong life. Physicians are not only given divine license to practice medicine, they are also mandated to use their skills to heal the sick. Failing or refusing to do so constitutes a transgression on the part of the physician.

In addition, all people are duty-bound to seek healing from a physician when they are ill and not to rely solely on divine intervention or faith-healing. They are charged with preserving their health when well, or restoring it when ill.

The physician's obligation to heal extends to the care of patients with contagious or communicable diseases if the potential risk to the physician is small. If the risk is substantial, physicians are not obligated to endanger their own lives.

NOTES

1. Tractate Sanhedrin, *Babylonian Talmud,* 73a.
2. Exodus 15:26.
3. Exodus 21:19.
4. Tractate Baba Kamma, *Babylonian Talmud,* 85a.
5. Fred Rosner, *Modern Medicine and Jewish Ethics,* 2d ed. (Hoboken, N.J. and New York: Ktav and Yeshiva University Press, 1991).
6. Immanuel Jakobovits, *Jewish Medical Ethics* (New York: Bloch, 1975).
7. Deuteronomy 3:3.
8. Deuteronomy 4:15.
9. Tractate Sanhedrin, *Babylonian Talmud,* 73b.
10. Moses Maimonides, *Mishneh Torah, Hilchot Rotzeach* 1:14.
11. Joseph Karo, *Schulchan Aruch, Choshen Mishpat* 426:1.
12. Joseph Karo, *Schulchan Aruch, Orach Chayim* 329:8.
13. Israel M. Kagan, *Mishnah Berurah* 329:19.
14. Abraham Z.H. Eisenstadt, *Pitchei Teshuvah, Choshen Mishpat* 426:2.
15. Terumot. end of chap. 8, according to *Ha'Amek Sheelah, She'iltot* 147:1.

16. Tractate Sanhedrin, *Babylonian Talmud,* 73a, according to *Agudat Aizov,* Derushim folio 3b and *Hashmatot* folio 38b.

17. David Zimra, *Responsa Radvaz,* Part 5 (Part 2 in *Leshonot HaRambam,* section 1, 508); *Responsa Radvaz* 3:627; and *She'iltot Radvaz* 1:52.

18. Leviticus 19:16.

19. Moshe Feinstein, *Responsa Iggrot Moshe, Yoreh Deah,* Part 2, no. 174:4.

20. Eliezar Y. Waldenberg, *Responsa Tzitz Eliezer,* vol. 10, no. 25:7.

21. Abigail Zuger, Steven H. Miles, "Physicians, AIDS, and Occupational Risk: Historic Traditions and Ethical Obligations," *JAMA* vol. 258, no. 2 (1987): 1924–28.

22. Jeremiah 21:9–10.

23. Tractate *Baba Kamma, Babylonian Talmud,* 60b.

24. Tractate *Baba Kamma, Babylonian Talmud,* 606.

25. Jeremiah 9:20.

26. Jakobovits, *Jewish Medical Ethics.*

27. American College of Physicians, Health and Policy Committee, and the Infectious Diseases Society of America: "The acquired immunodeficiency syndrome (AIDS) and infection with the human immunodeficiency virus (HIV)." *Annals of Internal Medicine,* vol. 108, no. 3 (1988): 460–69.

28. Association of American Medical Colleges, "Professional Responsibility in Treating AIDS Patients," *Journal Medical Education,* vol. 63, no. 18 (1988): 587–90.

29. George J. Annas, "Not Saints, But Healers: The Legal Duties of Health Care Professionals in the AIDS Epidemic," *American Journal Public Health,* vol. 78, no. 7 (1988): 844–49.

30. Ezekiel J. Emanuel, "Do Physicians Have an Obligation to Treat Patients with AIDS?" *New England Journal of Medicine,* vol. 318, no. 5 (1988): 1686–90.

31. David M. Laskin, "Treatment of Patients with AIDS: A Matter of Professional Ethics," *Journal Oral Maxillofacial Surgery* vol. 466, no. 9 (1988): 719.

32. Edmund D. Pellegrino, "Altruism, Self-Interest, and Medical Ethics," *JAMA,* vol. 258, no. 14 (1987): 1939–40.

On the Interface of Religion and Medical Science: The Judeo-Biblical Perspective

RABBI MOSHE TENDLER, PH.D.

INTRODUCTION

The Lord scrutinized all that He wrought and it was very good. [1]

The Lord said to (Adam and Eve): Be fruitful and fill the earth and *master it*! [2]

From all the trees of the Garden you may eat ... but of the Tree of Knowledge of Good and Evil you must not eat. [3]

LIMITATIONS OF SCIENTIFIC RESEARCH

Mastery of the natural world was granted to humankind. All of creation is to be in the service of mankind. There is no limitation on research that is designed to benefit mankind if the value system designed by G-d is honored. The forbidden Tree of Knowledge of Good and Evil is not a limitation on the search for knowledge but a proclamation that G-d defined Good and Evil. He did not leave it for man or society to redefine these absolutes that are the yardsticks by which the moral behavior of man and society is measured. This admonition is not intended to restrict the search for knowledge of our world, but only to assure that standards of ethical behavior are not violated. The license to "master" this world allows for topographic alterations and, when for our benefit, even exploitation of the animal kingdom, [4] but not the subjugation and violation of rights and privileges granted to every man and woman who are imprinted with the Divine Image. [5]

Science, and biblical ethics and theology, share several axioms:

1. There is order in the universe.
2. The human mind can perceive this order not only in broad constructs, but also in specific detail.

3. The unnatural is not innately bad. The unnatural or artificial, if sensitive to the Divine licensure under which we function, represents the fulfillment of the biblical commandment: "and master it."

These axioms deny the many superstitions and occult sciences that have plagued our world society since creation. That which the human mind recognizes as nonrational is not to be incorporated into our decision making. It is the world open to the scrutiny of the rational mind that is to be our field of operation. Alternative systems of medical science not subject to proof or disproof by carefully designed scientific protocol are not to be pursued. We are dependent on the personal protection of G-d who has approved rational medical science as proper intervention by man in time of sickness.

The command recorded in Exodus: "Heal he shall heal" [6] negates faith healing. When sickness strikes, the proper response is to seek healing through natural laws of sickness and health, in addition to relating to the Healer of all flesh through prayer. The duty to provide medical care is a personal obligation of every medical practitioner to whom the commandment: "You shall return it to him" (i.e., his lost health) is directed. [7] The duty to provide for medical care for all is imposed on nonphysicians as well by the commandment: "You shall not stand idly by" [8] which is interpreted as requiring the expenditure of funds to provide medical care for the indigent. This is the ethical basis for universal health insurance.

BIBLICAL ETHICS AND SCIENTIFIC METHODOLOGY

The moral code of Western civilization is based on principles of biblical ethics. These principles have served humanity well for over thirty-five hundred years in all countries under all social orders. Every society that attempted to substitute a value system other than one in consonance with traditional biblical ethics and morals failed to protect the weak and defenseless. Facism, communism, Oriental religions all share a common denominator—the degradation and exploitation of those who are powerless. The twentieth century has been a great challenge to the Christian and Moslem faiths. The two thousand-year experiment in modifying the Judeo-biblical heritage failed in its main mission—to humanize animal man. The Holocaust in Europe, the genocide in Rwanda, Biafra, and Bosnia perpetrated by faithful attendees at church and mosque is not an aberrant experimental result, but an undeniable proof that the experiment has not succeeded. The experimental design must now be changed in the hope of attaining the desired results.

APPLIED ETHICS

An ethical system can be judged only when it is seen in action, directing the decisions of its adherents. How does Judeo-biblical ethical tradition respond to the ethical dilemmas facing medical practitioners today? Response to the ethical issues at the beginning of life can serve to introduce this tradition to those unfamiliar with its teachings.

INFERTILITY AS AN ILLNESS

Give me children or else I die. [9]

The duty to heal applies to the "cure" of infertility. Defining infertility as an illness permits for the assumption of a modicum of risk in order to overcome the physiological barriers to successful gestation. It also obligates society to provide for such medical assistance to those in need.

PRO-CHOICE OR PRO-LIFE

He who spills the blood of man *within man* his blood shall be spilled. [10]

Abortion is tantamount to murder and can be sanctioned only when the life of the gestating mother is in danger. The great controversy when "humanhood" or "personhood" begins is not a medical-scientific debate, but rather one of religious traditions. The traditional biblical view assigns humanhood to an embryo at day forty. Abortion prior to day forty is prohibited except for medical concerns for the mother's health, while abortion after day forty cannot be permitted except to save the mother's life.

ASSISTED REPRODUCTIVE TECHNOLOGIES (ART)

The mastery of the reproductive process has led to the cure of many cases of the "illness of infertility." But new ethical dilemmas have arisen. The basic definition of "family" has been altered to substitute for the absence of genetic relationships. Donor insemination and ovum transplants introduce third-party genetic bloodlines into the husband/wife relationship. When the source of these gametes are close relatives, the biblical prohibition against incest is added to the question of adultery. Surrogacy, which separates genetic and gestational motherhood, raises the question of who is the real mother? Biblical tradition always assigned motherhood to the gestational mother, but the possibility of genetic, not gestational motherhood, could not be envisioned since the ovum was yet to be discovered in the nineteenth century. The purchase of ova from college coeds for the "going price" of $4,000 and the physiological cost of superovulation and ova harvest is of great ethical concern. Commodification of the human organism and risk assumption for others in return for financial remuneration would appear to violate fundamental biblical ethics. Biblical ethics considers surrogacy as a violation of the admonition not to subjugate man. Exploitation of a woman so that she will "rent" her uterus for nine months and assume the stresses of pregnancy and parturition must be seen at least as nibbling on the "forbidden fruit" of the Tree of Knowledge of Good and Evil.

The success in storing embryos for many years in the frozen state has added to our ethical concerns. If they are used after lengthy storage, there is a possibility of inversion of generation when an ovum fertilized in one generation is gestated by a descendant who, in effect, is giving birth to a grandparent! Biblical ethics is concerned with parent/child relationships; with clear distinction between generations born and unborn. Blurring these generational lines would seem to be morally indefensible.

MASTER OF THE DNA MOLECULE:
IS KNOWLEDGE AN ABSOLUTE GOOD?

1. The recent announcement (*Nature*, 23 February 1997) of the successful cloning of a sheep (not just splitting of a fertilized ovum during the early cleavage stages) is a dramatic reminder of the fantastic degree of mastery we have achieved over the molecule that carries the hereditary traits of all species. [11] Recombinant DNA research has been fueled by the spin-off from the international Genome Project. The scientific community has been overwhelmed by an avalanche of data and new technology to continue to increase this mastery of the molecule that is the determinant of the life of the cell, the organism and, therefore, of the species. The decision of most researchers to limit these modifications to somatic cells, not the germ plasm, is an action-oriented expression of deep concern for the dangers of eternalizing any genetic modification of a human genome. Somatic cells that have been altered will die with the organism. Germ cells are transferred to generations uncounted. It is as if scientists have by consensus classified germ-line experimentation as fruit of the Tree of Knowledge from which one should not eat.

2. Diagnosis without therapeutic potential: genetic probes are available for many genes that cause disease in late adult life such as Huntington's, Alzheimer's, multiple sclerosis, etc. Prenatal genetic analysis is available via

chorionic villi sampling, amniocentesis, embryo biopsy, and recently by the safe, noninvasive fetal sorting technique requiring but 5 cc of maternal blood during the ninth week of gestation. All of the almost two hundred genetic probes can be launched at these embryonic cells in an attempt to guarantee the "perfect child." Is this not a branch of the forbidden Tree of Knowledge, the fruit of which declares anyone with any discernible genetic defect as unworthy of living?

Until the therapeutic potential matches our ability to screen for defective genes, screening provides scientific ammunition to the proponents of eugenics who provided much of the impetus to Hitler's "Final Solution" that nearly destroyed the Jewish nation and with it tens of millions of people declared unfit to add their genes to the gene pool of the world. Indeed, the Human Genome Project is bringing about a resurgence of eugenics. As genetic technology becomes more accurate and more easily applicable, genetic paradigms of health and disease more widely accepted, genetic interventions will come to be expected and demanded. Eugenics is not medical genetics. Eugenic principles are concerned with manipulating population genetics to improve humanity by ridding the world of "bad genes." Medical genetics analyzes the genetic makeup of an individual to determine the nature of the disease in order to seek allopathic remedies. Indeed, medical genetics approaches eugenics when screening programs to prevent Tay-Sachs or cystic fibrosis or sickle cell anemia are introduced into schools and community centers. Medical genetics is concerned with preventing the birth of a "defective" child by counseling carriers not to marry each other. Eugenic principles dictate that a carrier never procreate so as to cleanse the human gene pool. Indeed, the Edwards/Steptoe research that led to in-vitro fertilization had two goals. Dr. Steptoe's interest was to permit a woman with blocked fallopian tubes to bear a child. Dr. Edwards' interest was to permit a woman or man with "defective genes" to raise a family using "approved" ova and sperm in accord with eugenic principles.

3. The ethics of screening and the right to know: the rule "what can be done will be done" applies to genetic screening. Private individuals can now locate research labs studying specific gene loci and for a fee request genetic probes. But should public policy be promulgated in favor of general screening for disease genes? A disturbing suggestion published in the highly reputable *New England Journal of Medicine* violates the fundamental ethical principle of "voluntary fully informed consent" in favor of "generic consent for genetic screening." [12] Recognizing that hundreds of new genetic screening tests will be introduced into routine clinical practice as a spin-off of the Human Genome Project, it will be impossible to do meaningful prescreening counseling about all available carrier tests. Information overload can make the entire counseling

process misleading or meaningless. Therefore, the authors suggest that "generic consent" be substituted for "fully informed consent." This suggestion, fraught with so much danger to the principle of patient autonomy so carefully cultivated since the 1970s, clearly summarizes the current dilemma. Mastering of the molecules of life is leading to mastery over those who have been given life. Economic concerns that are driving health care in America are searching the human genome for means of preventing disease. Genetic screening holds great promise for preventive medicine, but also great dangers to the ethical and moral standards of our society.

4. Value-laden counseling: genetic counseling is "value-laden." Fundamental principles of morals and religious tenets must enter the counseling equation. Where are there counselors well trained in medical genetics and well versed in the religious precepts of the major religions? Screening for a cancer gene or fragile-x syndrome is accompanied by a menu of alternatives; abortion, adoption, donor insemination, ovum transfer, sterilization—all value-laden with religious, ethical, and moral restraints. Surely screening without adequate counseling would be "cruel and inhuman punishment." Screening must wait until a cadre of multispecialty experts are properly trained.

5. Confidentiality and stigmatization: carriers of specific gene sequences are now experiencing discrimination in health insurance and in employment. The BRCA-1 and 2 gene that confers hereditary susceptibility to breast and ovarian cancer, or known genetic disease in family members has been the reason for rejection by health insurers. Mass screening would add many more reasons for discriminatory practices by insurers or employers whose health care premiums are negatively affected by the costly bills incurred by sufferers of genetic diseases. Indeed, they now request genetic probes of their choosing before issuing a multi-million-dollar policy. A mutated P-53 tumor suppressor gene, now easily detected by a genetic probe, may make an individual uninsurable! It is of historical and political significance that former Vice President Hubert H. Humphrey, who died of bladder cancer in 1978, had such a mutant gene in his cells. The violation of confidentiality that occurred with this announcement is concern enough, but the political consequence of knowing this information when deciding to accept the Democratic presidential nomination (only to lose to Richard Nixon) is of international import. Should every candidate for high office be required to submit to extensive genetic probing especially for the P-53 tumor suppressor gene?

Genetic disease is now a significant factor in social interactions. Genetic disease in the family impacts negatively on the marriage opportunities of all family members. Tay-Sachs and now cystic fibrosis screening is an accepted norm before a decision to marry is made. Children with challenging conditions—especially mental retardation that might have a genetic etiology—are "closeted" lest the chances for a good marriage of their siblings be diminished. If more extensive screening becomes routine, familial discrimination and social inequality will be a certain consequence.

6. Neuro-Calvinism: Genes and Behavior. During the last three years, claims have been published that specific genes control complex behavior patterns. A list of these gene-controlled behaviors include violence, hyperactivity, paranoid schizophrenia, alcoholism and drug abuse, sexual orientation, and reading disability. [13] These claims have put neurophysiology on a collision course with religion and with our legal system. If man is "coerced" by his gene spectrum to behave in a socially, religiously, legally unacceptable manner, he cannot be held responsible for his behavior either by G-d or by society. The existence of Free Will is a cornerstone of law and religion. To act as responsible moral beings, we must not be subject to physically or divinely imposed necessity. How does "genetic predestination" or Neuro-Calvinism allow for Free Will? The supposed conflict between science and religion has all but disappeared in our generation, only to be reawakened by behavioral genetics or sociobiology. Francis Crick, of double-helix fame, in a 1994 book, *The Astonishing Hypothesis: The Scientific Search for the Soul,* fuels this controversy by "attempting to wrest consciousness from the minds of the philosophers and place it in the hands of the scientists." [14] Witness the recent forensic review of the 1848 accident suffered by Phineas Gage in which an iron rod was driven through his brain by a dynamite blast; although he survived the injury with seemingly intact intelligence, his moral behavior was greatly altered as if a "moral faculty" was disrupted by the injury. Indeed a thesis seems to be gaining support that would affirm the accusation of ethicists that we are living in a "not-me" generation. Personal responsibility is rarely accepted for unethical behavior. Rather, the blame is transferred to genetic inheritance, mood modifying drugs, parental abuse, economic stress, black rage, inner-city fear syndrome, etc. How does the Judeo-biblical heritage view these coercive forces that impinge on our exercise of Free Will?

The "Cain Defense" was "Am I my brother's keeper?" [15] After killing his brother, Abel, Cain responded to G-d's rhetorical question: "Where is your brother Abel?" not by a denial but by a "not me" defense. I am not my brother's keeper, you G-d are! You gave me the ability to kill, you gave me the genes for violence. I am not responsible! This defense will not stand up in a heavenly court of law nor in our human legal system. The rebuttal to this defense was recorded earlier in the Bible when G-d admonished Cain for his irreverent altar-offering. "Sin waits at the threshold and it longs for you [and you for sin] but you can master it." [16]

Indeed, we have genetic traits as well as social forces that affect our thought processes and sway us to do evil. Each of us has his/her special temptations, unique moral blemishes. The nature of Free Will requires choices between good and evil and temptations to stray from the moral high ground. These inclinations to stray, be they genetically or sociologically determined, are controllable by ethical man. A rich man is tempted to exploit his workers. A poor man is tempted to steal from his employer. Neither wealth nor poverty coerces sinful behavior. G-d intended for rich and poor to be governed by the divine moral code designed for earth-bound man.

A sermonic tale that is recorded in the writings of one of the great commentaries on the Talmud speaks to the ethical dilemma posed by the realization that genetic traits do impact on ethical decision making. [17] A sheik sends out his best artist to the desert of Sinai to draw a portrait of the great Moses. Upon his return the sheik shows the portrait to his philosophers-physiognomists. They study the portrait and conclude that the face therein reveals a propensity for doing much evil. The righteousness of the great Moses as attested to by so many is thus challenged. The sheik cannot prove which of his subjects are incompetent, the artist or the philosophers. He feels compelled to make the trip himself. To his surprise he confirms the accuracy of the portrait drawn by his artist. Before concluding that his philosophers are charlatans, he requests an interview with Moses and relates to him the analysis of his philosophers. Moses responds by affirming the accuracy of both artist and philosophers. Indeed, Moses explains: "I do have genetic tendencies for moral, ethical lapses but by sheer force of my will I overpower these tendencies. That is why I earned the love of G-d and man."

This is an apocryphal tale that is the rebuttal of the Cain defense. We are our brother's keeper. We are not coerced to do evil, neither by genes nor by drugs nor by social forces. We need not join Crick's search for a soul. It lies within us and guides us in paths of righteousness.

NOTES

1. Genesis 1:31.
2. Genesis 1:28 (italics added).
3. Genesis 2:16–17.
4. Genesis 9:2.
5. Genesis 1:27.
6. Exodus 21:19.
7. Deuteronomy 22:2.
8. Leviticus 19:16.

9. Genesis 30:1.

10. Genesis 9:6.

11. A. E. Wilmut et al., "Viable Offspring Derived from Fetal and Adult Mammalian Cells," *Nature* 385 (Feb. 27, 1997): 810–13.

12. Sherman Elias and George J. Annas, "Sounding Board: Generic Consent for Genetic Screening," *New England Journal of Medicine*, vol. 330, no. 22, June 2 (1994): 1611–13.

13. *Science*, vol. 264, June 17 (1994): 1737.

14. Francis Crick, *Astonishing Hypothesis: The Scientific Search for the Soul* (New York: Scribner, 1994).

15. Genesis 4:9.

16. Genesis 4:7.

17. Israel Tifereth, tractate on marriages (Kiddushin), *Talmud.*

Healing and Being Healed: A Christian Perspective

EDMUND D. PELLEGRINO, M.D., M.C.A.P.

INTRODUCTION

Believers in a personal God must, if they are truly to live in the image of that God, be concerned for the afflictions of their fellow creatures. This is why solicitude for the sick has always been a grave obligation of the three major monotheistic religions. Their theological differences notwithstanding, Judaism, Islam, and Christianity share a common commitment to healing which has a common origin in the fatherhood of God, whose sovereignty over his creation is not that of the watchmaker, but that of the shepherd over his flock.

This essay focuses on healing as it is perceived by *a* Roman Catholic. It makes no claim to being *the* Christian, or *the* Roman Catholic perception. It seeks to express the author's sense of the scriptural origins and official church teaching about the obligation to heal and the meaning of healing conducted in the light of the Christian Gospels. It proceeds in three steps: First, an outline of the origins of the Christian perspective in the Old and New Testaments; second, an exposition of the Christian concept of healing; third, the practical implications of the Christian concept of healing for health professionals and the whole Christian community.

ORIGINS OF THE CHRISTIAN PERSPECTIVE

The roots of the Catholic Christian imperative to heal are deeply planted in the vivifying soil of the Jewish Bible and in the books of the Old Testament. God speaks to his people at Marah in the desert in these words, "I am Yahweh your healer." [1] He promises that if his people listen to his voice, follow his commands and do what is right, he will not afflict them as he afflicted the Egyptians. Through his prophets and patriarchs, Yahweh fulfills this promise many times.

Yahweh, on the appeal of Moses, heals Miriam of her skin disease and his people of the bites of snakes. [2] He cures King Hezekiah of a fatal illness [3] and through the angel Raphael, he instructs Tobias how to cure his father Tobits' blindness [4] and drive away the demon Asmodeus from his bride Sarah's bedroom. [5] Through Yahweh's healing power, Elijah restores life to the widow's son [6] and Elisha cures Naaman of his skin disease. [7] Even the ordinary physician effects his healing through God. [8] Many other instances of healing are found in the Jewish Bible and the Old Testament. [9]

The Christian imperative to heal and be healed is grounded in the healing episodes in the daily life of Christ as related in the Gospels. Next after his preoccupation with preaching the word of salvation, Jesus' most frequent activity in his earthly mission was healing the sick. The Gospels tell how multitudes flocked to Jesus throughout his public life and of how he healed many of their infirmities of body and mind:

> That evening after sunset, they brought to him all who were sick and those who were possessed by devils. The whole town came crowding round the door, and he cured many who were sick with diseases of one kind or another.... (Mark 1:32–34)

To this scene, which was repeated many times in the Gospels, we can add Jesus' own use of the parable of the Good Samaritan to instruct his followers. [10] Like the Samaritan, they were to care for the sick with solicitude even when they were strangers and even when it meant inconvenience and cost to the Samaritan. There is no need to recount Jesus' many miracles. His healing was always of both body and soul and always through the power conferred upon him by the Father. Jesus had a special affinity for those who suffered, for he knew that he too was to suffer. His own broken body was to be the way to the healing of mankind. Christ was thus the wounded healer, "the man of sorrows" prefigured in Isaiah, the one "... familiar with suffering, one from whom, as it were, we averted our gaze, despised, for whom we had no regard. Yet ours were the sufferings he was bearing, ours the sorrows he was carrying." [11] In the Talmud story, the Rabbi Yoshua ben Levi asked Elijah "When will the Messiah come?" Elijah told the rabbi to look for him at the gates of the city, binding his own wounds. He cared for his own wounds so that he would be ready to bind the wounds of others. [12] Elijah, like Jesus, was a wounded healer.

The Christian thus has two powerful images of Jesus—i.e., *Christus Medicus*, Christ the doctor, the healer, [13] and *Christus Patiens*, Christ suffering, [14] i.e., Christ the patient, the healer who knew suffering as no other has or could. This is a powerful set of images which fuse the physician's fragility with that of his patient, reminding him and her of their own mortality and need for healing. It combines Isaiah's suffering servant and Christ's healing servanthood. [15]

Despite the ubiquity of his healing, nowhere in the Gospels does Jesus offer a discourse on the nature of healing. His was not a ministry to doctors or philosophers. Healing was an act of love towards the sufferer, towards others with whom, as a human like them, he felt compassion. Jesus entered into the predicament of the sick in order to relieve, console, care, and cure. For Jesus healing needed no justification in philosophy or theology. Healing was a promise the Father had made to his people. Jesus healed through his fidelity to that promise.

By his healing, Jesus changed the ancient world's notion of illness as odium, as punishment for sin, or as a sign of inferiority. His healing showed that sickness was not a disgrace, the sick and lepers were not to be shunned: "I was sick and you visited me. Inasmuch as you do this unto one of the least of my brethren, you have done it unto me." The sick person now had a preferential position, and it became a duty of the entire Christian community to care for all its sick and poor. [16]

It is out of the powerful example of Jesus' life that healing became for Christians a special ministry, a vocation, a call from God to serve God and one's fellows. For Christians healing is, therefore, not an occupation; it is a calling, a way of life and of salvation for those who are professed healers. It is this image of Christ the healer that inspired the establishment of hospitals in the early church and spawned so many orders of religious men and women and monastic communities devoted to the care of the sick. [17] Healing and care of the sick are woven intimately into the fabric of Christianity from its beginnings. The thread is continuous from God's first encounter with his people to the present moment, and it will continue into the future until the end of human existence.

A CHRISTIAN PHILOSOPHY OF HEALING

If we seek a philosophy of Christian healing, we can draw it only inferentially from sources other than the Gospels. The Gospels teach directly by exhortation, parable, and example, not by argument. A Christian philosophy of healing must begin with God, the creator of human life, the giver of a precious gift, the creator of a human soul united with a body. Those who receive this gift inherit the duties of stewardship—duties to preserve the well-functioning of the soul, body, and mind, never to abuse them, to heal them when they are ill and healing is possible, and to care for and sustain them when cure is not possible.

On this view, self-abusive behaviors—overeating, indolence, smoking, abuse of alcohol, failure to rest, exposing oneself to disproportionate risks and stress—are violations of a sacred stewardship. On this stewardship view, it also follows that there is a strong prima facie obligation to seek out and accept effective treatment when illness occurs. Health, like life itself, is a precious gift. Not to sustain health, or to refuse effective treatment, is, on the face of it, an act of ingratitude and infidelity to the duties of stewardship.

But life itself and bodily and mental health are not absolutes. They may be risked for the good of others when risk is unavoidable, e.g., to save the lives of others, to serve others better, and especially if our station in life requires risks. Physicians treating those with contagious diseases, firemen or policemen doing their duties, or soldiers defending their countries are called upon by their special roles to risk even the gift of life for the welfare of others. Reckless risk to life is not condoned, but neither is survival as the supreme good. Death need not be artificially prolonged when treatment is futile and death is inevitable. When the outcome of treatment is so dubious or marginal as to be highly improbable, and the physical, emotional, and fiscal burdens are out of proportion to the benefits, treatment can be refused or discontinued. This balance between the probability and gravity of the burdens of treatment (physical, emotional, fiscal, social) and the benefits to the patient must be struck prayerfully, carefully, and never with intent to usurp the sovereignty of God, the creator of life.

Healing in the Christian sense is always more than body repair. Healing an illness is often a restoration of our relationship with God. Jesus said to those he healed, "Because of your faith, it shall be done to you." (Matt. 9:28) Christian healing gives us hope and a strengthened faith that God loves us and that this love will sustain us in the chaos and turmoil of illness. We know that no matter what happens, God will not abandon us or leave us to face our perils alone. He will give us the grace to come closer to him through our illness. It is human to reject suffering, to hope for a miracle, and even to pray for it. It is a gift of grace to know, through illness, the limits of mind and body and find wholeness of spirit in the experience. When this occurs, illness itself becomes a healing experience.

If the miracle we pray for does not come, it does not mean God has abandoned us. Every time Christ healed, even miraculously, it was the spiritual healing that counted. Physicians today can perform technical miracles like helping the blind to see and the lame to walk. But this is only part of true healing. Christian healing is holistic in the best sense: it strives to heal the body, but it also recognizes that any serious illness involves a spiritual crisis, a confrontation with the questions of God and our relationship to him. In illness, one may reject that relationship, but no one can ignore it, not even the atheist or agnostic.

The whole Christian community is called to imitate Christ—whether we are health professionals, family members, friends, or sick, ourselves. All of us are called to offer solicitude for the sick, to comfort them in their suffering, to sustain their hope, to be present to them. When they are dying, we can, and must, help the sick to experience God's love for them even when all the world seems alien, when they feel depressed, guilty, or hostile. The sick will always ask Job's questions: "Why, Lord? Why me? Why now?" None of us can answer those questions. But we can comfort and console when it becomes clear, as it did to Job, that God does not owe us an answer.

As Cardinal Bernardin so eloquently said during his own encounter with pancreatic cancer:

> Our distinctive vocation in Christian health care is not so much to heal better or more efficiently than anyone else; it is to bring comfort to people by giving them an experience that will strengthen their confidence in life. The ultimate goal of our care is to give to those who are ill through our care a reason to hope. [18]

This goal of hope is a direct contradiction to the despair that so often leads patients, their families, and physicians to see euthanasia and assisted suicide as the only remedy. This despair is at the heart of the spiritual crisis of terminal illness. When one confronts one's own finitude as a fact, here and now and inevitable, hope cannot survive without a personal God who has promised not to let us face our perils alone. Pain relief is not the major reason for consciously accelerating death. It is depression, despair and abandonment unrestrained by a source of hope beyond medical technology, even friends or family.

Christian healing, while it provides spiritual sustenance for hope, does not ignore healing the body or relieving pain. We are embodied spirits, not angels. Not to use pain medication optimally is a failure in healing and a form of moral and legal malpractice. Too many Christian physicians fear moral sanction if death accidentally results or the patient becomes addicted. Clinically these are unlikely outcomes in patients already receiving high doses of opiates. In any case, they can be justified by proper reference to the moral rule of "double effect." [19] Death as an unintended consequence of intrinsically good acts of pain relief is not evil if it is not intended and does not depend on the act of killing to achieve its purpose.

True healing also means relief of suffering, the emotional, spiritual, and highly personalized response to the predicament of illness. For the Christian, healing can occur even as the patient is dying and suffering, right up to the last moments. That is why hastening death by euthanasia is neither compassionate nor beneficent. [20] Christian physicians, friends, and family members are called in the order of charity to sustain, help, comfort, and be present for the sick person. They must heed Isaiah's words which so keenly described the loneliness, the averting of our eyes from the suffering servant. [21]

Christian presence is not the callow judgmental presence of Job's friends. Job's friends, at first, sat silently with him for seven days and seven nights. After that, they succumbed to the temptation of pious logorrhea, with sanctimonious explanations of why God visited sickness on Job. They began to construct syllogisms to prove Job had sinned. They were really hiding their own terror. If Job, the just man, could be visited with such suffering, how much more vulnerable were they? So they talked compulsively and defensively like so many visitors to the sick do. God and Job, himself, chided them for their wordiness. [22] Christian healing means giving of oneself, being truly present, listening, sharing the burden, accepting the dying person not as the alien being he feels himself to be, but as still a full member of the human community. The Christian task to is help the sufferer live his/her last days well, with hope in God and not as a victim of despair, guilt, and rejection.

Christians cannot give each person the answer to the meaning of his or her suffering. That meaning can only come from each person's own confrontation with God, in his or her own way, in the context of his or her own life story. It is not the abstract meaning of suffering in general we seek, but its meaning for this person before us now. For some, suffering will mean reconciliation with God; for others reconciliation with self, family, or friends; for some, a deepening understanding of the meaning of their lives. [23] Our Christian faith tells us that we are not alone, that God will not abandon his children, that no life is without meaning. Who are we to say what suffering means in someone else's life? Who can possibly know the transforming power of our lives on others even when we seem most powerless? We must allow for the operation of the Holy Spirit even when our lives appear meaningless to us.

Christian healing requires compassion—feeling something of the sick person's burdens as our burdens, literally suffering along with him or her. This is not the distorted compassion that impels others to urge or suggest euthanasia or assisted suicide. That is compassion gone awry, compassion more directed to the anguish of those who attend and live with the dying person than the person suffering. Compassion is a normal human emotion in the face of suffering. But it is not itself a justifying principle or a virtue. Compassion gets its moral status by the nature of the end to which it is directed, not from assuaging the feelings of those who experience it. Compassion deals more with suffering than pain. By communicating our genuine sharing of the burden, we can help, heal, and comfort others and, incidentally, often heal ourselves. "Compassion" cannot sanction killing the suffering person or helping him to kill himself.

Christian healing is healing centered on respect for the human person, for his and her inherent dignity as a creature of God. Every human has dignity and that dignity cannot be lost through illness, debility, disfigurement, or dying. Our dignity is rooted in the fact that we are made in the image of God. [24] This does not mean we are God, but rather that he has given humans a special place in the cosmos. This dignity cannot be taken from us and it entails respect by others. Only imputed dignity is lost. This is the dignity attributed to us by those who attend us in our sufferings. The observer's disaffection for illness, fear, and even repugnance give a clear message which says, "I don't want to be that way." This robs the patient of his imputed, but not his actual, dignity. If the sick person feels undignified and asks for that dignity to be restored by death, the indictment is often against us, the living, who have robbed him of his dignity. It cannot be an indictment of the dying person's inherent dignity as a child of God, which can never be lost.

Suicide and euthanasia are not ways to recapture dignity. The patient cannot confer dignity on himself, nor can the doctor confer it on the dying patient. It is not theirs to confer. Everyone dies with his inherent dignity intact. Loss of dignity is only in the eye of the beholder. Those who accept their own finitude can transform the lives of those who witness their dying. This can be their parting gift to those they love.

THE CHRISTIAN PERSPECTIVE IN PRACTICE

What differences does the Catholic Christian perspective on healing make in the lives of patients and health care professionals?

To begin with, certain models of the healing relationship, the relationship between health professionals and patients will be more acceptable than others; some will be totally unacceptable. This is a crucial matter at present when the traditional models are being drastically altered by societal, political, and economic forces. [25] A Christ-inspired relationship could never be encompassed within a contract, for example. Contracts are legalistic, protective agreements between people who do not trust each other. They minimize both trust and commitment. They are not valid when either party is under compulsion to enter the contract, as is the patient who is by the nature of being ill vulnerable, anxious, dependent, and exploitable. Moreover, there is no way a patient can anticipate all the potential hazards which he might wish to guard against. Indeed, a strict binding contract could hamper decision making to such a degree as to be counterproductive.

Likewise, a Christian healing relationship could never be based in any of the market-inspired models, e.g., a commodity transaction with the physician as entrepreneur, case manager, fundholder, rationer, or any of the other noxious metaphors of industry, business, or commerce which are so popular with economists, managed care executives, policymakers, and marketing specialists. Healing within the Christian context is inconsistent with the profit-driven care, trading of patients as assets, or liabilities in mergers and buy-outs, or with "cherry-picking," i.e., the deselection or dropping of really sick patients in favor of the healthy, more profitable young premium payer.

The healing relationship cannot be like that of the mechanic to one's automobile, or of the biologist to his subject of study, or of the technician to her machinery. The only morally viable model would be the covenantal model. This is the special relationship of a sacred promise and trust between one who is ill and in need of help and one who offers himself or herself as a healer. The Christian healer—and indeed any true healer—is one who is committed primarily to the welfare of the sick person rather than to his own. This suppression of self-interest is the mark of a true profession. [26]

A second practical consequence of a Christian healing imperative is to make healing a vocation, a sacred calling to imitate Jesus' solicitude and his examples of healing. Healing, therefore, is not to be simply an occupation, a way of making a living, fashioning a career, gaining power, prestige, or profit. Rather, healing must become a call to a station in life, one with special obligations to others, a way to our own salvation and the salvation of those whom we treat.

A third consequence is the way the Christian perspective modifies the principles of medical ethics. Each principle is transmuted by charity, the ordering Christian theological virtue. I have expanded on this idea in detail elsewhere. [27] Let me summarize here: beneficence would be more than non-maleficence, more than avoiding harm or even doing good. It means doing good even when it means sacrifice of self-interest. Autonomy would focus on respect for persons and their dignity as creatures, not on some absolute freedom or license to do with our lives what we please. Respect for persons would, indeed, emphasize self-governing decision making. But our freedom as creatures of God is always within the constraints of ethical and moral determinants derived from Scripture, tradition, church teaching, and the study of ethics.

Justice, on this view, would be reshaped as charitable justice—justice, as someone has said, with the "blindfold" removed—justice modulated by love, not strictly weighed, but justice favoring the disadvantaged whenever possible. This is the sense of the official Roman Catholic Church position of a "preferential option" for the poor. In health policy, it would mean equity in distribution of essential services regardless of ability to pay. It entails universal accessibility to health care without discrimination. On this view, health care becomes an obligation of the whole Christian community because charitable justice recognizes a moral claim on all of us by the sick, disabled, poor, and rejected members of our society.

Charitable justice also requires *pro bono* work on the part of all the healing professions. It also means their technical knowledge and skill could never be proprietary. Rather, they are stewards of the knowledge they possess because others need that knowledge to flourish as humans. On this view, a medical education is a privileged access to medical knowledge, dissection of human bodies, autopsies, care of patients when in medical school, etc. In all of these parts of a medical education, the usual "rights" of sick persons are modified to present a new generation of students to become healers. On this view, justice also imposes on the professional the duty of advocacy for the poor who do not have access to health care; when necessary political action to influence policymakers on behalf of the disadvantaged is also a community and professional obligation. Charitable justice may also require refusal to obey unjust laws or practices that harm the sick person in any way.

The whole Christian community, therefore, stands indicted when there are members of our society whose sufferings go underserved or are deprived of health care. Health care is not a privilege but an obligation a Christian and a good society owes its citizens. To be sure, each of us is called to care for his or her own health. But when our fellow humans fail in this obligation, we must nevertheless respond to their needs. There is no room on the Christian view for vindictiveness or punishing those who fail in their stewardship of their bodies by denying care when they need it.

A society loses moral status in relation to the amount of suffering and deprivation it tolerates in its citizens. There is today—at a time when our affluence as a nation is at its height—a startling disparity in access to medical and health care. Christians have an obligation to work for alleviation of this disparity. A Christian society by definition must be a society based in charitable justice. More explicitly, Christians must be prepared themselves to make the sacrifices necessary for just distribution of health care. Otherwise, the example of Jesus' healing ministry will be little more than a myth without meaning for our individual daily lives.

On a Christian view of healing, the divided loyalty, the appeal to the physician's self-interests through financial incentives, the deceptions of the gag rule, and the secrecy of the contractual arrangements of managed care would be morally intolerable. The same could be said of members of the Christian community who profit from the plight of sick persons as investors, managers, or executives of managed care organizations. Practices at the moral margins, like ownership of for-profit health care facilities, equipment, or laboratories are suspect. Physicians who see patients, or make rounds with Mammon as their preceptor, hardly qualify as Christ-inspired healers. The moral harms of certain managed care arrangements is yet to be fully explored or deplored.

Clearly, Christ-inspired healing would also recognize the responsibility of health professionals who reject euthanasia and assisted suicide to become expert in palliative care. To heal while someone is dying and suffering is an awesome responsibility. We must treat the sufferer without glorifying suffering. This entails some diagnosis of why *this* patient is suffering, and entering the unique experience of his or her illness. Dying patients are not interested in a general explanation of suffering. Suffering arises in a complex interaction among a variety of causes—feelings of guilt, unworthiness, rejection and alienation by and from the well, being a financial, emotional, and physical burden to others, feeling guilty by spending one's estate on futile treatment. To these are added the immediacy of one's finitude, hostility to God, and the sense of being unjustly punished, which can be found even in usually devout patients. Those factors interact in each person in combinations unique to his/her life story.

If we are to heal suffering, it is our task, through listening, to discern and differentiate these causes of suffering in *this* patient, to unravel the interplay of those complex factors, and to relieve them by providing the emotional, communal, and familial support that healing wounded humanity so acutely demands.

It would be presumptious to try to give every patient the full meaning of his suffering. But we can help each patient to understand the roots of his suffering and try compassionately to remove them. Our task is to heal within the spiritual ambience suited to *this* patient, here and now. This is true healing, to "make whole again" in the fullest sense, even when the consummation of earthly life is unavoidable and imminent.

CONCLUSION

Healing the sick has a special meaning and a special obligatory force for Christians, since it is so firmly rooted in both the New and Old Testaments. Christians are called to nothing less than the imitation of ineffable models, Jesus and Yahweh himself.

The practical implications of fidelity to Christ's imperative to healing and solicitude for the sick are clear. They influence the models of patient care we choose, the methods of financing and distributing health care in society we support, and the way we interpret and apply the usual principles of medical and health care ethics as well as the way we care for the incurable and the dying.

None of us can be so prideful that we think we can fulfill Jesus' teaching to perfection. Even Mother Teresa, who came as close as any human can, did not claim more than an attempt to come as close as possible to what the Gospels teach. Nonetheless, each of us, within whatever legitimate constraints life imposes, is called to be solicitous for the sick among us and in society. For health professionals this call is our ordained way of life and salvation.

NOTES

1. Exodus 15:16. (All Scripture citations are from the *New Jerusalem Bible* [New York: Doubleday, 1990]).
2. Numbers 12:13–15, Numbers 21:6–9.
3. 1 Kings 20:1–2, Isaiah 38:4–6.
4. Tobit 11:11–15.
5. Tobit 8:1–3, Tobit 6:1–9.
6. 1 Judges 17:20–22.
7. 2 Kings 5:3–14.
8. Sirach 38.
9. Exodus 15:26; Numbers 12:13–15; Numbers 21:6–9; 2 Kings 20:1–2; 1 Kings 17:20–22; 2 Kings 5:3–14.
10. Luke 10:29–37.
11. Isaiah 53:3–4.
12. Cited by Henri J. M. Nouwen, *The Wounded Healer* (Garden City, New York: Image Books, 1979): 81–82.
13. St. Peter Cryologus, *Collectio Sermorum,* Cl. 0227, M, SL 24, Sermon 50, Line 61.
14. Augustinus Hipponensis, *Enarrationes in Psalmos,* CL 0283, SLL 40, Psalmus: 130 Par: Line 18.
15. Isaiah 53.
16. Henry E. Sigerist, *Civilization and Disease* (Ithaca, New York: Cornell University Press, 1944): 69.

17. Darrell W. Amundsen, "Medicine, Society and Faith," *Ancient and Medieval World* (Baltimore: The Johns Hopkins University Press, 1996): 127–57, 175–221.

18. Joseph Cardinal Bernardin, *The Gift of Peace: Personal Reflections* (Chicago: Loyola Press, 1996): 5.

19. Orville Griese, *Catholic Identity in Health Care: Principles and Practice* (Braintree, Mass.: The Pope John Center, 1987).

20. Edmund D. Pellegrino, "The False Promise of Beneficent Killing" in *Regulating How We Die,* ed., Linda L. Emanuel (Cambridge, Mass.: Harvard University Press, 1998): 71–91.

21. Isaiah 53:3.

22. Pellegrino, "The Trials of Job: A Physician's Meditation," *Linacre Quarterly,* vol. 56, no. 2 (May 1989): 76–88.

23. Miguel De Unamuno, "The Tragic Sense of Life" in *Men and Nations,* trans., Anthony Kerrigan (Princeton, N.J.: Princeton University Press, Bollingon Series, LXXXV, 4, 1972): 222.

24. Genesis 1:26.

25. Pedro Lain Entralgo, *Doctor and Patient,* trans., Frances Partridge (New York: McGraw-Hill, 1969).

26. Pellegrino and David Thomasma, *For the Patient's Good: The Restoration of Beneficence in Health Care* (Oxford: Oxford University Press, 1987).

27. Edmund D. Pellegrino, "Agape and Ethics: Some Reflections on Medical Morals from a Catholic Christian Perspective," *Catholic Perspectives on Medical Morals,* eds., John P. Langan and John C. Harvey (Dordrecht: Kluwer Academic Publishers, 1989): 277–300.

A Catholic Christian Perspective on Early Human Development

REV. J. D. CASSIDY, O.P., PH.D.

The Gospel of life (the good news to the people for every age and culture). It is precisely for this life that all the aspects and stages of human life achieve their full significance. [1]

The Gospel of God's love for man, the Gospel of the dignity of the person, and the Gospel of life are a single and indivisible Gospel. [2]

A distinguished contemporary physician, theologian, and medical ethicist has identified certain fundamental and believed truths relative to Catholic medicine and especially to the unborn patients entitled to welcoming, caring, and sharing life. Among these are "that God has created human beings; we are made in his image; all human beings share in his love; and the Spirit is given to us to guide and inspire us on our pilgrimage to our everlasting home, heaven." [3]

Respect for human life and the dignity of the human person from the earliest moments of conception to natural death are the keystones of Roman Catholic ethics and bioethics. This essay will:

1. Address the nature and origin of this moral conviction in the Jewish and Christian Sacred Scriptures and church documents and the biological continuum of human embryological development;
2. Define the responsibilities of family, church, and society; and
3. Relate both to the formulations of universal human rights through application of the Catholic Consistent Ethic of Life.

"IMAGO DEI": CREATED IN GOD'S IMAGE AND LIKENESS

According to Catholic belief, the initial and complex human fertilization reaction begins each personal life history. Therefore, the human being must be respected—as a person—from the first instant of his or her existence. [4] Of all visible creatures, only man is able to know and love his or her creator. [5] The Catholic Church teaches that persons alone are called to share, by knowledge and love, in God's own life. It was for this end that she or he was created, and this is the fundamental reason for his or her dignity. [6] Being created in the Image and Likeness of God, [7] the human individual possesses the dignity of a person who is not just something, but someone. [8] The value of the newly created life springs from her or his being the *Imago Dei*, from her or his having, in the likeness to the Creator, an orientation toward placing oneself in a relationship to him. [9] The awesome gift given at human fertilization begins the adventure of a new life, and each of its capacities requires time, a rather lengthy time, to find its place and to be in a position to act, [10] during the subsequent months of gestation.

Catholics formally enter this new life through the new birth of baptism. In the ancient tradition of clothing with the white garment during the rite of baptism of infants, the new Christian is reminded: "See in this white garment the outward sign of your new Christian dignity. With your family and friends to help you by word and example, bring that dignity unstained into the everlasting life of heaven." [11] The religious roles of parents and godparents, and also their stewardship duties are brought out more clearly in the rite itself. "The human body shares in the dignity of the Image of God; it is a human body precisely because it is animated by the spiritual soul and it is the whole human person that is destined to become, in the Body of Christ, the temple of the Spirit." [12] Christian parents will recognize that this practice of the baptism of infants also accords with their role as nurturers of the life that God has entrusted to them. [13]

From the initial steps of each pilgrimage of life, the newly conceived human zygote should be treated as a human person. [14] By his reason, man recognizes the voice of God which urges him to do good and avoid what is evil. [15] Everyone is obligated to follow this law, which makes itself heard in conscience and is fulfilled in the love of God and neighbor. Living a moral life bears witness to the dignity of the person. [16] Each new member of the human community is welcomed as a unique gift on a personal journey of human embryology, protected by God, through responsible parents and the family as the sanctuary of life. [17] From the first Christian century, ecclesiastical law taught parents in the Didache: "You shall not kill the embryo by abortion and shall not cause the newborn to perish." [18]

Civilized societies guard the most vulnerable developing members of their human community as biological subjects of protected human rights. [19] Guided by the law of nature and its natural inclinations and proclivities, even pagan Visigoth law would execute and blind parents guilty of abortion and infanticide. All parents as heirs and guardians of the gift of life share, as moral agents and as a gift, the task of bringing new human beings into the world. [20] Catholic Christians and many Churches of the Book share the Judaic conviction of the centrality of the revered gift of life and the nature of man himself ". . .as something splendid or divine as a creature with freedom and dignity." [21] What is at stake is nothing less than the idea of the dignity and worth of each human being.

The mystery of each new creation at human conception, the belief that the human soul is created by a direct act of God at the time of fertilization and that each person is unique and irreplaceable, shapes the Roman Church's doctrine that the human embryo is a human being. [22] Fertilization represents the scientifically and morally logical place to draw the line between what is and is not human life. [23]

Recently, the Pontifical Academy for Life, international experts on the identity and status of the human embryo, including biologists, physicians, philosophers, theologians, and jurists, confirmed that the moment of fertilization marks the constitution of "a new human organism equipped with an intrinsic capacity to develop itself autonomously into an individual adult." [24] "From a biological standpoint, the information and the development of the human embryo appears as a continuous, coordinated and gradual process from the time of fertilization, at which a new human organism is constituted, endowed with the intrinsic capacity to develop by itself into a human adult." [25] "The most recent contributions of the biomedical sciences offer further valuable empirical evidence for substantiating the individuality and developmental continuity of the embryo." [26] "The ethical exigency of respect and care for the life and integrity of the embryo, demanded by the presence of a human being, is motivated by a unitary conception of man (body and soul) whose personal dignity must be recognized from the beginning of physical existence." [27] "The theological perspective, beginning with the light which revelation sheds on the meaning of a human life and on the dignity of the person, supports and sustains human reason in regard to these conclusions, without in any way diminishing the validity of contributions based on rational evidence." [28]

"Therefore, the duty of respecting the human embryo as a human person derives from the reality of the matter and from the force of rational argumentation, and not exclusively from a position of faith." [29] "From the juridical point of view, the core of the debate on the protection of the human embryo does not involve identifying earlier and later indices of humanity which appears after insemination, but consists rather in the recognition of fundamental human rights by virtue of the presence of a human being." [30] This learned academy reaffirmed that "above all, the right to life and to physical integrity from the first moment of existence, in keeping with the principle of equality, must be respected." [31]

Several faith communities concur that advances in human biology have come to prove that "in the zygote arising from fertilization, the biological identity of a new human individual is present." [32] It is the individuality proper to an autonomous being, intrinsically determined, developing in gradual continuity. [33] The covenant between God and man is interwoven with reminders of God's gift of human life. [34] It can be welcomed properly and protected against the many attacks to which it is exposed and can develop in accordance with what constitutes authentic human growth. [35]

Human life is believed to be sacred because from its beginning it involves the creative action of God, and it remains forever in a special relationship with the Creator. God alone is the Lord of life from its beginning until its end. [36] Thus, the sacred and inviolable value of life and the right to live of every human person were confirmed in the recent papal encyclical letter on human life. [37]

Human dignity rests above all on the fact that a person is called to communion with God: a personal divine vocation. This invitation to converse with God is addressed to man as soon as he comes into being. [38] The dignity of the developing child is proclaimed by the psalmist and by the prophet in Divine Revelation: "For you formed my inmost being." [39] "Before I formed you in the womb, I knew you, and before you were born I consecrated you." [40] Thus, the life of every individual, for her or his unique beginning is part of God's plan, [41] and the incomparable value of each developing human being are both accepted Catholic beliefs.

Pope John Paul II teaches that the life of every individual, from its beginning, is part of God's plan. [42] He recalls the greatest value and equal worth of every developing human life and every person, [43] and the indisputable recognition of the value of life from its very beginning is celebrated in the New Testament in the meeting between the Virgin Mary and Elizabeth and between the two children whom they are carrying in the womb. [44]

From biblical dawn we are obligated to protect human life. Genesis 9:5 teaches clearly that "from man in regard to his fellow men I will demand an accounting," interpreted through the millennia as reverence and love for every human life. [45] The fact that life belongs to God and not to the human being gives it that sacred character which produces an attitude of profound respect: "A direct consequence of the divine origin of life is its inviolability, its untouchability, that is, its sacredness." [46] Man's life comes from God; it is a gift, this

Image, and this imprint, a sharing in this breath of life. God, therefore, is the sole Lord of this life: man cannot do with it as he will. God himself makes this clear to Noah after the flood. The biblical text is concerned to emphasize how the sacredness of life has its foundation in God and in his creative activity, "for God made man in his own image." [47]

THE CHURCH AND MODERN GENETICS

Pope John Paul II acknowledges the extraordinary results obtained by science, e.g., the progressive discovery of a human genetic map and the increasingly precise information on the sequence of the genome ... in support of the church's doctrine on the sacredness, inviolability, and grandeur of human life. [48]

Through its Charter of the Rights of the Family (1983) the Vatican teaches the inviolability of members of our species: Human life must be absolutely respected and protected from the moment of conception. Modern genetic science ... has demonstrated that, from the first instant, the program is fixed as to what this living being will be: a man, this individual man, with his characteristic aspects already well determined. [49] This teaching is confirmed by recent findings of biological science which recognize that in the zygote resulting from fertilization, the biological identity of a new human individual is already constituted. [50] Further, this Vatican declaration affirms that: "Respect for the dignity of the human being excludes all experimental manipulation or exploitation of the human embryo." [51] The practice of keeping alive human embryos *in vivo* or *in vitro* for experimental or commercial purposes is totally opposed to human dignity. [52]

THE CHURCH AND THE EARLIEST STAGES OF THE HUMAN CELL CYCLE

The initial patterns of the preimplantation stages of human and mammalian development have been researched and characterized by Saunders, [53] O'Rahilly and Muller, [54] Moore, [55] Blandau, [56] Anderson et al., [57] Burger and Weber, [58] and Braude et al. [59] They have detailed the striking organization and the earliest patterns of steps in the human journey at the level of the fine structures of the zygote and blastomeres. Specifically, they have observed the functional complexes between cells during predictable cleavage divisions of the zygote and the spatial, numerical, and temporal polarity and differentiation of the trophoblast and inner cell mass of early and later blastocysts formed during the first weeks of human embryogenesis. Such observable and awesome unfolding of each newly conceived person's genetic program is a scientific testimony to the Divine Creator's providential design of the early journey of each *Imago Dei.*

There is a continuum of changing developmental, patterned stages beginning from conception to the formation of the zygote through precise cleavages of the two-cell, four-cell, eight-cell morula stage blastomeres during the personal journey through the fallopian tube—to the implantation of the growing blastocyst in the posterior wall of the mother's uterus. This developmental process traces each step in the genesis of human rights that inhere in each person. From the earliest stages of human development, genetic exactness of distinct human cleavage polarities, and numerical, spatial, and temporal patterns are present. In their absence, early human developmental handicaps, arrests, or disabilities arise.

FROM BEGINNING OF LIFE RESEARCH VERSUS THE TECHNOLOGICAL IMPERATIVE

Many researches are assembling the genetic map of the individual human's biological traits through the coordinated work of the Human Genome Project. The results will enable persons to trace their hereditary patrimony and anticipate their genetic handicaps and disabilities. Concomitantly, preimplantation genetic diagnosis is now possible as early as three days of embryonic age when the cleavage embryo is composed of only four to eight cells. [60] It is claimed that one or two of the blastomeres may be removed for genetic analysis, e.g., of the cystic fibrosis trait, without adversely affecting the remaining cells of the developing embryo. This diagnostic technique has eugenic potential. It was pursued experimentally by its applications to an individual human embryo who developed subsequently into a healthy baby. Moral evaluations of experimental human procreation depend on the moral principle which affirms that what is technically possible is not always morally right. [61] From the advent of experiments in human embryo duplication and the prospect of research into cloning, the Vatican insisted that unscrupulous scientists who "venture into a tunnel of madness" must be regulated. [62] This echoed the insistence of the papal encyclical that the end does not justify the means—if science is to be morally good. [63]

CONSISTENT HUMAN RIGHTS AND RESPONSIBILITIES

Developing human embryos and fetuses at the beginning of their personal journey, and waiting to be born, are safeguarded by the comprehensive Catholic moral analogy, the Consistent Ethic of Life. [64] This is a timely synthesis of natural rights theory clearly protective of persons during their earliest development. It is firmly rooted in the biblical sanctity and equal dignity of each person, and the inalienable natural right to live with human dignity of every human being—the "basic right" [65] of the unborn. A derived moral principle follows; namely, that any unjust attack on a developing innocent human being is unethical. Whatever the violence, whether discrimination against the gender or anticipated quality of the new life, abortive destruction, or experimental manipulation, it is judged to be a grave injustice opposed to the rights of inviolability and indiscardability of the new person.

Such guiding Catholic beliefs are germane to moral evaluation of the new reproductive technologies. They help to focus the church's constraints against the misuse of research in science and technology. They foster advocacy for the renewed culture of life and intelligibility by opposition to infanticide, convenience and induced abortion, cloning, and nontherapeutic embryo and fetal experimentation. Concern for those waiting to be born also helps to strengthen permanent marriage and responsible parenthood by clarifying parental stewardship obligations of begetting, nurturing, and educating of children. They are the great gifts of life entrusted by the Creator to creative, loving parents. Many persons of Gospel faith are called to be responsible stewards of their most vulnerable offspring, guided and guarded as biological subjects of human rights. [66] In the current controversies about the right to life, members of the Catholic Church and other biblical faith communities strongly oppose destruction of the developing innocent for any reason. Making abortion a "choice" is an usurpation of the absolute dominion God has over the universe and all its parts. Violations of human rights are at the basis of the church's opposition to renewed eugenic practices based upon genetic endowments, economics, all forms of directed social evolution, and political theory. [67]

ORIGIN OF HUMAN RIGHTS IN HUMAN DIGNITY

Many of the claims of global human rights derive from Judeo-Christian faith and the philosophical traditions of natural law and natural rights. Fifty years ago scholars of the Book with Judeo-Christian convictions, like Jacques Maritain, Rene Cassin, and Charles Malik, were among the founding committee of the Universal Declaration of Human Rights adopted by the UN General Assembly in 1948." [68] As for the "key" in which the various rights were to be "harmonized," the Universal Declaration belongs to a family of postwar rights instruments that accord their highest priority to human dignity. In its preamble, the Declaration states: "Whereas recognition of the inherent dignity and of the equal and inalienable rights of all members of the human family ... Whereas the peoples of the United Nations have in the Charter reaffirmed their faith in fundamental human rights, in the dignity and worth of the human person ..." [69] Natural human rights are reinforced also by the recent agreements of the European community in the Convention on Human Rights and Biomedicine of the Council of Europe. [70]

In this fiftieth anniversary of the Declaration, and the firm grounding of the rights inherent *in* every person, more international consistency is needed to link the proclamation with its realization in practice. All need to be freed by the monitum of the "Gospel of Life" papal encyclical against the lingering contradiction threatening the entire culture of human rights. Despite the nobility of the various declarations of human rights and the many iniatives inspired by them, the right to life is still being violated, especially at the most vulnerable moments of existence, i.e., the moments of birth and death. [71] Pope John Paul II describes the paradox of global growing moral sensitivity to the value and dignity of every individual human being, on the one hand, and a tragic and chilling repudiation in practice on the other. This threat to life reminds us of the biblical context of Cain's question: "Am I my brother's keeper?" [72] Articles 1 and 3 of the accepted United Nations' Universal Declaration ought to guarantee affirmative replies: "All human beings are born free and equal in dignity and rights" and "Every one has the right to life, liberty, and security of person"! [73]

CONCLUDING RELIGIOUS REFLECTIONS

The American Catholic bishops and the pope have emphasized repeatedly the manifold mystery involved in the journey from the onset of human life. The church's commitment to human dignity inspires an abiding concern for the sanctity of human life from its very beginning and with the dignity of marriage and of the marriage act by which human life is transmitted. The church's defense of life encompasses the unborn and the care of women and their children during and after pregnancy. The church's commitment to life is seen in its willingness to collaborate with others to alleviate the causes of high infant mortality and to provide adequate health care to mothers and their children before and after birth. The church has the deepest respect for the family, for the marriage covenant, and for the love that binds a married couple together. This includes respect for the marriage act by which husband and wife express their love and cooperate with God in the creation of a new human being. Marriage and conjugal love are by their nature ordained toward the begetting and education of children. Children are really the supreme gift of marriage and contribute very substantially to the welfare of their parents. Parents should regard as their proper mission the transmission of human life and education of those to whom life has been transmitted. Parents are, thereby, cooperators with the love of God the Creator, and are, so to speak, the interpreters of that love. [74] Scientists and doctors must not think that they are lords of life, but rather its experts and generous servants." [75]

The elements of divine vocation, human journey, and personal pilgrimage in the Gospel of Life are present already in the revelation of the earliest biblical books and, indeed, written in the heart of every man and woman, and have echoed in every conscience from the beginning. In summary, from the time of creation itself . . . each can be known in its essential traits by human reason. [76] For Christians, too, the instruction of the Book of Deuteronomy's invitation rings out so helpfully: "See I have set before you this day life and good, death and evil . . . I have set before you life and death, blessing and curse: therefore choose life, that you and your descendants may live." [77] We pilgrim people, the people of life and for life, take our steps in confidence towards a promised "new heaven and new earth;" [78] and we look to *her*, who is for us "a sign of sure hope and solace" ". . . mother of the living, to you do we entrust the cause of life." [79]

DEDICATION

In grateful tribute to the memory of His Eminence, Joseph Cardinal Bernardin's forty-four years of service to human life in all of its profound mysteries. He was an architect and articulator of the principles of the Consistent Ethic of Life, and cofounder of the national initiative, the Catholic Common Ground Project. In the words of his lifelong friend and associate, "Always a unifier, he reached out to leaders in the Catholic Church and those of other faiths because he wanted common ground to become holy ground." [80]

NOTES

1. Pope John Paul II, *Evangelium vitae (The Gospel of Life)* (Boston: Pauline Books and Media, 1995): 1.

2. Pope John Paul II, *Evangelium vitae,* 2.

3. John Collins Harvey, "An Introduction to the Biological and Medical Aspects of In Vitro Fertilization" in *Gift of Life,* Edmund Pellegrino, John C. Harvey, and John P. Langan, eds. (Washington, D.C.: Georgetown University Press, 1990): 47.

4. Sacred Congregation for the Doctrine of the Faith, *Donum vitae (Instruction on Respect for Human Life in Its Origin and on the Dignity of Procreation)* (Vatican City), I: 1.

5. Genesis 1:27; Genesis 2:24; Mark 10:2–12.

6. *Catechism of the Catholic Church*, (San Francisco: Ignatius Press, 1994): 357.

7. Genesis 1:26; Genesis 1:27; Genesis 5:1, 2; Genesis 9:6; Romans 8:29; 1 Corinthians 11:7; 2 Corinthians 4:4; Colossians 1:15; Colossians 3:10; Hebrews 1:3.

8. *Catechism of the Catholic Church*, 357.

9. Joseph Cardinal Ratzinger, "Reconciling Gospel and Torah: The Catechism of the Catholic Church," *Origins* 23 (1994): 621.

10. Sacred Congregation for the Doctrine of Faith, *Acta Apostolicae Sedis (Declaration on Procured Abortion)*, (1974): 66.

11. *The Rites of the Catholic Church* (New York: Pueblo Publishing Co., 1976): 1.

12. *Catechism of the Catholic Church*, 364.

13. *Catechism of the Catholic Church*, 1251.

14. Sacred Congregation for the Doctrine of Faith, *Donum vitae*, I: 1.

15. Pastoral Constitution on the Church in the Modern World, *Gaudium et spes* (1961): 16.

16. *Catechism of the Catholic Church*, 1706.

17. Pope John Paul II, *Evangelium vitae*, 92–94.

18. Didache 2, 2: *Schol.* 248: 148.

19. Benedict Ashley and Albert S. Moraczewski, "Is the Biological Subject of Human Rights Present from Conception?" in *The Fetal Tissue Issue* (Braintree, Mass.: The Pope John Center, 1994): 33–59.

20. *Universal Declaration of Human Rights*, (New York: United Nations, 1948): Preamble.

21. Leon R. Kass, *Toward a More Natural Science* (New York: The Free Press, 1985).

22. Kevin D. O'Rourke and Philip Boyle, eds., *Medical Ethics: Sources of Catholic Teaching* (St. Louis: Catholic Health Association of the United States, 1989): 3.

23. Pontifical Academy for Life, "The Embryo: When Human Life Begins," *Origins* 26 (1997): 662–63.

24. Pontifical Academy for Life, "The Embryo."

25. Pontifical Academy for Life, "The Embryo."

26. Pontifical Academy for Life, "The Embryo."

27. Pontifical Academy for Life, "The Embryo."

28. Pontifical Academy for Life, "The Embryo."

29. Pontifical Academy for Life, "The Embryo."

30. Pontifical Academy for Life, "The Embryo."

31. Pontifical Academy for Life, "The Embryo."

32. Sacred Congregation for the Doctrine of the Faith, *Donum vitae*, I: 1.

33. Fiorenzo Cardinal Angelini, *Charter for Health Care Workers*, (Vatican City: Pontifical Council for Pastoral Assistance to Health Care Workers, 1995): 35.

34. *Catechism of the Catholic Church*, 2260.

35. Pope John Paul II, " '*Centesimus Annus*': Encyclical on the 100th Anniversary of '*Rerum Novarum*'," *Origins* 21 (1991): 1.

36. *Catechism of the Catholic Church*, 2258.

37. Pope John Paul II, *Evangelium vitae*, I: 11.

38. Pastoral Constitution on the Church in the Modern World, *Gaudium et spes* (1961): 19, 1.

39. Psalm 139:13 (NAB).

40. Jeremiah 1:5 (NAB).

41. Pope John Paul II, *Evangelium vitae,* 44.

42. Pope John Paul II, *Evangelium vitae,* Introd. 2.

43. Pope John Paul II, *Evangelium vitae,* 45.

44. Pope John Paul II, *Evangelium vitae,* 39–41.

45. Fiorenzo Cardinal Angelini, *Charter for Health Care Workers,* 43.

46. Pope John Paul II, *Evangelium vitae,* 39.

47. Genesis 9:6 (NAB).

48. Sacred Congregation for the Doctrine of the Faith, *Donum vitae,* I: 1.

49. Sacred Congregation for the Doctrine of the Faith, *Donum vitae,* I: 1.

50. *L'Osservatore Romano* (25 November 1983): 4b.

51. Sacred Congregation for the Doctrine of the Faith, *Donum vitae,* I: 4.

52. Sacred Congregation for the Doctrine of the Faith, *Donum vitae,* I: 1.

53. John W. Saunders, *Developmental Biology: Patterns, Problems, Principles* (New York: Macmillan, 1982).

54. Ronan O'Rahilly and Fabiola Muller, *Developmental Stages in Human Embryos* (Washington, D.C.: Carnegie Institution of Washington, 1987).

55. Keith L. Moore, *The Developing Human: Clinically Oriented Embryology* (Philadelphia: Saunders, 1988); *Before We Are Born: Basic Embryology and Birth Defects* (Philadelphia: Saunders, 1989).

56. Richard J. Blandau, *The Biology of the Blastocyst* (Chicago: University of Chicago Press, 1971).

57. Everett Anderson, P.C. Hope, W.K. Whitten, and Gloria S. Lee, "In Vitro Fertilization and Early Embryogenesis: A Cytological Analysis," *Journal of Ultrastructure Research* 50 (1995): 231–52.

58. Max Burger and Rudolf Weber, eds., *Embryonic Development,* 1 (New York: Alan R. Liss, 1982): 69–85.

59. Peter Braude, Virginia Bolton, and Stephen Moore, "Human Gene Expression Occurs between the Four- and Eight-Cell Stages of Preimplantation Development," *Nature* 332 (1988): 459–61.

60. Peter Braude, Virginia Bolton, and Stephen Moore, "Human Gene Expression."

61. Richard A. McCormick, S.J., "Blastomere Separation: Some Concerns," *Hastings Center Report* 24 (1994): 14–16; U.S. Bishops, "Ethical and Religious Directives for Catholic Health Care Services," *Origins* 24 (1994): 457; Albert S. Moraczewski, O.P. "Cloning Testimony: National Bioethics Advisory Commission in Washington, D.C., March 13, 1997," *Ethics and Medics* 22 (1997): 3–4.

62. *L'Osservatore Romano* (23 October 1993).

63. Pope John Paul II, *Veritatis Splendor,* "The Splendor of Truth" (Boston: St. Paul Books & Media, 1993).

64. Joseph Cardinal Bernardin, "A Consistent Ethic of Life: An American-Catholic Dialogue," *Origins* 13 (1993): 491; "Health Care and the Consistent Ethic of Life," *Origins* 15 (1995): 36; "The Consistent Ethic: What Sort of Framework?" *Origins* 16 (1986): 345–50.

65. Pope John Paul II, *Centesimus annus, Origins* 21 (1991): 27.

66. Benedict Ashley, O.P. and Albert S. Moraczewski, O.P., "Is the Biological Subject of Human Rights Present from Conception?" in *The Fetal Tissue Issue: Medical and Ethical Aspects* (Braintree, Mass.: The Pope John Center (1994): 33–59; Pope John Paul II, *Evangelium vitae*, IV: 91.

67. Pope John Paul II, *Evangelium vitae*, I; Council of Europe: "Convention for Protection of Human Rights and Dignity of the Human Being with Regard to the Application of Biology and Biomedicine: Convention on Human Rights and Biomedicine," *Kennedy Institute of Ethics Journal* 7 (1997): 277.

68. Mary Ann Glendon, "Reflections on the UDHR," *First Things* 82 (1998): 23–25.

69. "Universal Declaration of Human Rights (1948)," *First Things* 82 (1998): 28.

70. F. William Dommel, Jr., and Duane Alexander, "The Convention of Human Rights and Biomedicine of the Council of Europe," *Kennedy Institute of Ethics Journal* 7 (1997): 259.

71. Pope John Paul II, *Evangelium vitae,* 18.

72. Genesis 4:9 (NAB).

73. United Nations General Assembly, "Universal Declaration of Human Rights" (New York: 10 December 1948).

74. U.S. Bishops, "Ethical and Religious Directives for Catholic Health Care Services", *Origins* 24 (1994): 456–57.

75. Pope John Paul II, *To the Pontifical Academy of Sciences,* 21 October 1985 in *Insegnamenti VIII/2,* 1081.

76. Pope John Paul II, *Evangelium vitae,* II: 44.

77. Deuteronomy 30:15–20; Pope John Paul II, *Evangelium vitae,* I: 28.

78. Revelation 21:1 (NAB).

79. Dogmatic Constitution on the Church, *Lumen gentium,* in *Documents of Vatican II* (New York: Guild Press, 1966): 68.

80. Kenneth Velo. "An Instrument of His Peace", *Extension* 91 (1996): 4; Joseph Cardinal Bernardin, "Called to be Catholic: Church in a Time of Peril", *Origins* 26 (1988): 165–70; Daniel Pilarczyk, "A Common Ground for Jews and Christians", *Origins* 16 (1987): 815–16.

Epilogue: Religion and Bioethical Discourse

Edmund D. Pellegrino, M.D., M.C.A.P.

The "dialogue" in this volume between Jewish and Christian perspectives in medical ethics takes place at a time when the dominant orientation of bioethics has become secular, nonreligious, or even antireligious. But it also occurs at a fortuitous moment in the history of moral philosophy when secular ethics, itself, is also under critical scrutiny. Until thirty or so years ago, medical ethics still retained some remnant of its centuries-long connections with religion. But when, in the 1960s, medical ethics became the subject of more formal philosophical inquiry, it quickly became part of the dominant project of modern moral philosophy, i.e., the pursuit of an ethics free of religion and metaphysics. This has been the aim of secular philosophy since the Enlightenment. [1,2]

On this post-Enlightenment view, moral arguments based in religious traditions, Scripture, or church teachings are inadmissible in ethical discourse. Believers are, of course, free to follow the precepts of their own religions, so long as they do not impinge on the freedoms of others or use religious arguments in political debate. In a morally pluralistic, democratic, and diverse society, human reason constrained by religious belief, or by moral authority beyond human determination, must be a private affair. This is the credo of the most influential voices in the emergence of contemporary "bioethics" (Beauchamp and Childress, [3] The Belmont Report, [4] the President's Commission [5]).

To be sure, the voices of religiously based ethicists have not been absent. Jakobovits, [6] Rosner, [7] Franck, [8] and others have represented the Jewish tradition, while Ramsey, [9] McCormick, [10] and Gustafson [11] have spoken for Christian ethics. There have been areas of concordance between these religiously based perspectives and secular bioethics, largely on decision-making procedures but not on substantive ethics. On the "human life" issues, especially abortion, euthanasia, assisted suicide, embryo research, reproductive technologies, cloning of humans, preimplantation embryo diagnosis, surrogate parenthood, etc., the incommensurability between religious and secular ethics has grown. As biologists probe more deeply into, and gain greater control over, human genetics, and as moral philosophy grows ever more pragmatic, utilitarian, and antifoundational, the metaphysical and religious questions cannot be avoided. [12] One must either deny meaning to such questions as secularists do, or grapple with them as religious and theological ethicists must do.

Protagonists of an exclusively philosophical ethics take different views of religion. Some are indifferent, simply excluding it as mythology in the more deprecatory sense of that word. Others are more tolerant, yet condescending. They grant the value of religion as a psychological prop but banish it from ethical discourse or policy formulation. Others are more frankly negative. Like Nietzsche, they see religion as a baleful influence, seducing people into docility and corrosion of independent thought. In the last decade, however, this high tide of secular bioethics has begun to turn, for several reasons.

First, many have found philosophical ethics, at least utilitarian and principle-based ethics, too abstract and too impoverished of concrete detail to capture the full complexity of the moral life. As a result, much attention has focused on casuistry, narrative, feminism, experience, practice, dialogue, consensus, and public opinion as alternative ways to determine right and wrong, good and bad. These alternatives purport to engage a wider and richer range of elements in the moral life, often including the religious elements even if doctrinal elements are denied.

Second, others argue that the diversity of religious, ethnic, or cultural perspectives in our modern, democratic societies precludes agreement on substantive ethics. A more process-oriented ethic seems more suitable. On this view, ethics must concentrate on how we make decisions more than on the actual decisions we make. Whatever laws, regulations, public opinion, and committees can agree upon must substitute for stable definitions of right or wrong. The emphasis is on "rights," due process, and individual freedom to decide what is good or evil. A variety of contractarian, communitarian, dialogical theories are proposed to deal with the diversity of moral opinion by seeking "consensus."

Finally, also in the last decade, in America at least, the antifoundationalist *Zeitgeist* has entered moral philosophy. On this view, propounded by so-called "postmodernists" and "deconstructionists," reason, itself, is suspect as well as any overarching theory of ethics. Autonomous reason, the cornerstone of secular bioethics, is itself now under attack. [13] With metaphysics and religion already gone, there is little left to support the structure of moral philosophy except praxis, consensus, or emotivism. Moral skepticism, relativism, or pragmatism have assumed normative status. [14] As a result, the gap between secular and religious bioethics is growing wider daily.

However, for the very reasons just adduced, religion is being invoked as a means of recapturing meaning in ethics and as an antidote to the inescapable frustration of moral skepticism. The realization is growing that there is no avoiding the "deeper" questions. These are the questions about human nature, the meaning of human life, existence, and destiny. These are, and remain, the questions religion and metaphysics have always examined. They provide the ultimate sources that give morality its substance. Polls repeatedly show that the majority of Americans believe in religion and God. There is renewed interest in the power of prayer in healing. [15] The question now before bioethics is how philosophical and theological ethics can and ought to relate to each other both in ethical discourse and in public debate.

The essays in this volume outline the perspectives of two of the world's most influential religions, i.e., Judaism and Christianity. Both are monotheistic. Both believe in a personal God, one who continues his interest in the world he has created. Both possess authoritative sources for right and wrong that are grounded in the Scriptures and in authoritative teachers who interpret those Scriptures as God's word. For both Christianity and Judaism, religion, reason, and faith interlock to give a full picture of the moral life.

Judaism (at least Orthodox Judaism) and Roman Catholicism (at least among those faithful to the Magisterium) are firmly grounded in an ultimate source of morality, i.e., the word of God as enunciated in the Holy Scriptures. In Judaism, there is the centuries-old tradition of talmudic and rabbinic interpretation of the meanings of the law. In Catholicism, the long tradition of teaching by councils, synods, the popes, and theologians serves to explicate and interpret Scriptures. Judaism and Catholicism are, therefore, foundational in their ethical teachings. Each provides an overarching vision of the world and of morality. Each is, therefore, in direct confrontation with the antifoundational thrust of contemporary ethics.

Catholicism, further, is traditionally a natural law ethic, one which derives its ethics from a philosophical anthropology and theory of human nature with its telos in this world and the next. Roman Catholicism is thus unapologetically foundational, both in its theology and philosophy. Indeed, among ethical systems, Catholicism often is at the most extreme pole from the current antimetaphysical biases of contemporary bioethics.

Orthodox Judaism and Roman Catholicism—and, to varying degrees, the more conservative Protestant and Muslim denominations—also stand clearly outside the perimeters of contemporary bioethics. These religions are true "alternatives" to modernism and postmodernism. They are not, and cannot be, simply variants of current secular theories of ethics. They counter antifoundationalism with foundations, relativism and subjectivism with moral authority, and moral hubris with moral humility. To the dictum, "Nothing in ethics is absolute," they reply that some things ought never be done.

These polarities are more obvious every day as the debates in bioethics become more widespread in public discourse. People are now beginning to see the importance of religion in bioethics as the source of ultimate meaning absent from modern ethical theories. Those who hope for some compromise between these polarities miss the full implications of the differences in prelogical presuppositions, moral epistemology, and conceptual content of the secular and the religious perspectives. Increasingly, the fundamental choices seem to be between a strictly theological ethics, a thorough-going secular one, or some interdigitation of philosophy and theology.

Engelhardt has argued strenuously that ethics can only be done in communities that share fundamental moral values. [16] This would preclude effective ethical discourse between religious and nonreligious ethicists. Engelhardt's virtue is to follow his line of reasoning to its logical conclusion. Yet, his conclusion, if it were applied rigorously, would make ethical discourse difficult or impossible even within communities with shared values. All of us belong to overlapping value systems, some of which are in conflict with each other. When dealing with our internal conflicts, we eventually resolve them at least in part. At some point, we do choose a course of action and follow it. We would otherwise be paralyzed in a state of velleity.

But as we move from the pivot of our own internal perception of the good to the wider world of the good as perceived by others, the disjunctions between our personal notion of the good and that of others become manifest. Without a common conception of the good for human beings, there is little chance of agreement on morality, which is ultimately a search for, and statement of, the good for humans. Failure of agreement seems to be the inevitable future for medical ethics and for moral philosophy more generally. Yet humans are social and political animals. Their moral and ethical convictions cannot be held in isolation from each other. Humans must live in community if they are to survive and flourish.

The way increasingly followed is that of a minimalistic procedure-based ethics which purportedly eschews questions of substantive ethics, except in communities of "shared values." But in our polyglot contemporary society, such communities are becoming progressively less likely to exist than ever before. The other extreme of agreement on a unifying ethics based in a universally accepted overarching religion and metaphysic seems equally unlikely short of the Second Coming. For some of us, one alternative is to elaborate an updated and reinvigorated natural law ethic with its roots in those things common to all humans as humans.

This refurbished natural law ethic could be the common ground between secular and religious medical ethics at least, if not the whole of moral philosophy. It could center on the ends internal to medicine which, in turn, are grounded in the phenomena of illness and healing—phenomena common to humans as humans. [17] The metaphysical and religious questions would remain. The search for a better definition of foundations would continue. Antifoundationalism is, after all, itself, a form of foundationalism since it is an overarching theory, albeit a nihilistic one.

There is at least the possibility that secular bioethics will push the envelope of nonfoundationalism to its perimeters and that its supporters may realize that the only protection against the destruction of all reason is a return to a metaphysics of some sort and then, perhaps, even to a religious foundation for ethics. Not many may take this route, but appreciating its possibility may, in the end, possibly allow for a better *modus vivendi* between the religious and the secular views of medical ethics specifically and moral philosophy generally.

In this respect, Stephen L. Carter's defense of the legitimacy and necessity for religious argument in civil debate deserves careful attention. He makes a good case for the "habit of civility" while defending the right of persons with religious beliefs to dissent in democratic societies from laws they find offensive to their beliefs. He uses Martin Luther King's crusade for civil rights as an example of the kind of assertion of religious morality that would be suppressed if we adhered to a strict disenfranchisement of religious argument in public debate. [18]

If Carter is right about the place of religious moral argument, and if the shortcomings of antifoundationalism and secular bioethics are as clear as they seem to be, there is promise for more productive dialogue between and among secular and religiously based bioethics in the future. The alternative is an increasing widening breach and lack of civility, portending serious divisions in ethical perspective, the end result of which will be not only strife but isolation of each of us in increasingly narrower communities of shared values.

With so many Americans committed to religious belief in their personal lives, and with the issues raised by bioethics touching so intimately on those lives, it is inconceivable that the current disenfranchisement of religion in bioethical discourse can endure. The polarities between the religious and nonreligious perspectives, and within these perspectives themselves, will no doubt continue. But as the shortcomings of a secularistic perspective become ever more manifest, the playing field promises to be more level.

This is critical in the policy arena where legislation on matters concerning bioethics affects the lives of all. Whereas, until now, secularism has dominated the debate, religion can no longer be disenfranchised. This will make things more difficult. But the difficulties cannot be wished away by either the believer or the secularist.

NOTES

1. Alasdair MacIntyre, *After Virtue: A Study in Moral Theory* (Notre Dame, Ind.: University of Notre Dame Press, 1981): 51–61.

2. H. Tristram Engelhardt, Jr., *The Foundations of Bioethics,* 2d ed. (New York: Oxford University Press, 1996).

3. Tom L. Beauchamp and James F. Childress, *Principles of Biomedical Ethics,* 4th ed. (New York: Oxford University Press, 1994).

4. National Commission for the Protection of Human Subjects of Biomedical and Behavioral Research, *The Belmont Report: Ethical Principles and Guidelines for the Protection of Human Subjects of Research [Department of Health, Education, and Welfare Publication OS 78-0012]* (Washington, D.C.: U.S. Government Printing Office, 1978).

5. President's Commission for the Study of Ethical Problems in Medicine and Biomedical and Behavioral Research, *Deciding to Forego Life Sustaining Treatment* (Washington, D.C.: U.S. Government Printing Office, 1983).

6. Immanuel Jakobovits, *Jewish Medical Ethics* (New York: Bloch Publishing Company, 1959).

7. Fred Rosner, *Jewish Bioethics* (New York: Sanhedrin Press, 1979).

8. Isaac Franck, ed., *Biomedical Ethics in Perspective of Jewish Teaching and Tradition* (Washington, D.C.: College of Jewish Studies of Greater Washington, 1980).

9. Paul Ramsey, *Ethics at the Edges of Life* (New Haven, Conn.: Yale University Press, 1978).

10. Richard A. McCormick, *Notes on Moral Theology 1965–1980* (Washington, D.C.: University Press of America, 1981).

11. James A. Gustafson, *The Contributions of Theology to Medical Ethics* (Milwaukee, Wisc.: Marquette University Press, 1975).

12. Gilbert C. Meilaender, *Body, Soul, and Bioethics* (Notre Dame, Ind.: University of Notre Dame Press, 1995).

13. Richard Rorty, *Objectivity, Relativism, and Truth* (New York: Cambridge University Press, 1991).

14. Stephen Toulmin, "The Primacy of Practice: Medicine and Post-Modernism in Philosophy of Medicine and Bioethics" in Ronald A. Carson and Chester R. Burns, eds., *A Twenty Year Perspective and Critical Appraisal* (Dordrecht: Kluwer Academic Publishers, 1997): 41–53.

15. Dale A. Mathews with Connie Clark, *The Faith Factor* (New York: Viking Press, 1998).

16. H. Tristram Engelhardt, Jr., *The Foundations of Bioethics.*

17. Edmund D. Pellegrino and David C. Thomasma, *For the Patient's Good: The Restoration of Beneficence in Health Care* (New York: Oxford University Press, 1988).

18. Stephen L. Carter, *Dissent of the Governed: A Meditation on Law, Religion, and Loyalty* (Cambridge, Mass.: Harvard University Press, 1998).

Index

A

abortion
earliest Christian teachings on, 128–29
exceptions to ban on, 28–30, 60, 108
fetal tissue transplants, 63–64
Jewish laws on, 39
Maimonides on, 29–30
objections to restrictive moral code, 65–66
partial-birth, bill to veto, 25
reasons for, 30, 32
active euthanasia, 34, 47, 49. *See also* euthanasia
adultery, abortion after, 32
affliction, definition of, 77
AIDS patients, 103. *See also* contagious diseases, treating patients with
American College of Physicians, 103
American Medical Association Council on Ethical and Judicial Affairs, 103
Anderson, Everett, 131
antivitalism, 65–66. *See also* non-vitalism; vitalism
assisted reproductive technologies (ART), 108–9
Association of American Medical Colleges, 103

Astonishing Hypothesis: The Scientific Search for the Soul, The (Crick), 112
At the Will of the Body (Frank), 89–90
Auerbach, Shlomo Z., 20
"Auschwitz, Morality and the Suffering of God" (Sarot), 88
autonomous reason, 140
autonomy
disposing of one's body, 46
focus of on respect/dignity, 122–23
limits to individual, 27
loss of, 69
role of patients', 20
axioms, 106–7

B

baptism, 128
Beauchamp, Tom, 139
Belmont Report, The, 139
beneficence, 122
Bernardin, Joseph, Cardinal, 60, 62, 119, 135
best-interests model of patient care, 92
biblical ethics, 107
Blandau, Richard, 131
Bleich, David, 19, 27
Bolton, Virginia, 131
Braithwaite, R. B., 11